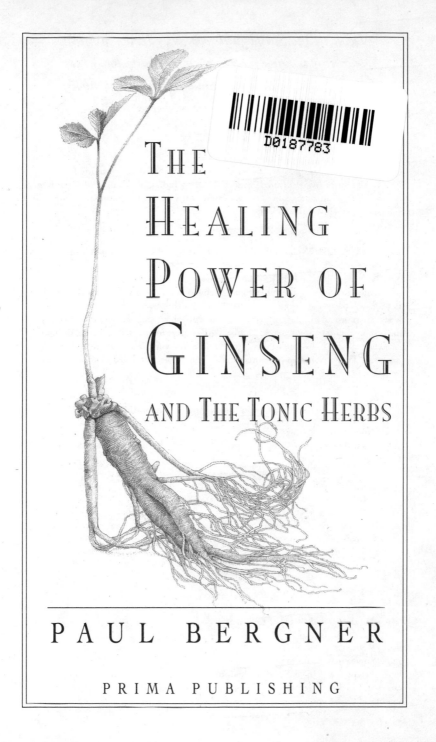

THE
HEALING
POWER OF
GINSENG
AND THE TONIC HERBS

PAUL BERGNER

PRIMA PUBLISHING

Dedicated to Satya Ambrose, ND, L.Ac., my first teacher of Chinese medicine, and to the doctors at the Open Gate Clinic in Portland, Oregon, who embody the spirit of service in Chinese medicine.

PRIMA PUBLISHING and colophon are trademarks of Prima Communications, Inc.

WARNING—DISCLAIMER: Prima Publishing has designed this book to provide information in regard to the subject matter covered. It is sold with the understanding that the publisher and the author are not liable for the misconception or misuse of information provided. The author and Prima Publishing shall have neither liability nor responsibility to any person or entity with respect to any loss, damage, or injury caused or alleged to be caused directly or indirectly by the information contained in this book. The information presented herein is in no way intended as a substitute for medical counseling.

Library of Congress Cataloging-in-Publication Data

Bergner, Paul.
 The healing power of ginseng & tonic herbs : the enlightened person's guide / Paul Bergner.
   p. cm.
 Includes index.
 ISBN 0-7615-0472-9
 1. Ginseng—Therapeutic use. 2. Tonics (Medicinal preparations) I. Title.
 RM666.G49B47 1996
 615'.323687—dc20   96-15742
                        CIP

96 97 98 99 00 AA 10 9 8 7 6 5 4 3 2 1

Printed in the United States of America

How to Order:
Single copies may be ordered from Prima Publishing, P.O. Box 1260BK, Rocklin, CA 95677; telephone (916) 632-4400. Quantity discounts are also available. On your letterhead, include information concerning the intended use of the books and the number of books you wish to purchase.

CONTENTS

SCIENTIFIC RESEARCH ON GINSENG

THE TONIC HERB FAMILY

HOW TO USE GINSENG AND THE TONIC HERBS

PRODUCTS: HOW TO BUY GINSENG AND THE TONIC HERBS

Acknowledgments

I would like to acknowledge the following contributions to this book.

For granting interviews: Mark Blumenthal, Bill Brevoort, Howie Brounstein, Richo Cech, Andrew Gaeddert, Feather Jones, Gary Schweedock, Dr. Jill Stansbury, Dr. Michael Tierra, Dr. Sharol Tilgner, Jonathan Treasure, and several others in the ginseng industry who asked not to be named.

For their previous books on Chinese tonic herbs, all of which I consulted while writing this book: Dan Bensky, Steven Foster, Ron Teeguarden, and Dr. Michael Tierra.

For editorial assistance at Prima: Alice Anderson, Leslie Yarborough, and especially Carol Venolia, who rescued several sections from a stranglehold of bad grammar and cloudy thinking.

For ginseng samples: Feather Jones and HerbPharm.

For personal support: Marian Barone, Aaron Bergner, Dr. Pao-Chin Huang, Feather Jones, and Dr. Doug Terry.

I ask the indulgence of those many practitioners of Oriental medicine whose knowledge and understanding is greater than my own should they find faults in this book. I ask them to accept this as an offering to introduce this beloved system of medicine to the American public.

LIST OF TABLES

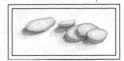

INTRODUCTION

North Americans in the 1990s are in a different state of health than any previous population group in the world. No people in the past have endured such unremitting stress, consumed so much junk food, taken so many pharmaceutical drugs, gotten so little sleep, abused so many stimulants, or lived in such a toxic environment as do Americans today. Even the slaves in ancient Greece and Rome had 115 holidays a year. Americans are overfed but undernourished. Chronic fatigue, immune deficiency, depression, anxiety, and stress-related disorders are rampant. As a nation, we are becoming chronically run down.

Conventional medicine has nothing to offer the exhausted patient. Its powerful therapies may temporarily suppress a symptom but will do nothing to restore overall energy and balance to the system. Even Western traditions of herbalism and natural healing were developed mainly on robust peasant and farmer populations who were well fed on lean organic meat and fresh vegetables. Western natural therapies aim to reduce the ill-effects of too much food rather than to restore vitality to a depleted system.

· This run-down state of the population is one reason for the growing popularity of ginseng (pronounced jín-sing), the most famous of the tonic herbs from China. Ginseng sales are among the fastest-growing categories of herb sales in the U.S., with products now available even in most drug stores, supermarkets, and pharmacies. However, most Americans are unaware of how to use ginseng. They do not understand its properties, know its contraindications and side effects, or know the difference between Asian and American ginseng or other herbs mislabeled as "ginseng." They also do not understand how to buy ginseng in a marketplace filled with questionable and outright fraudulent products. I will explain all these points in this book.

Ginseng is only the most famous of a whole category of Chinese tonic herbs, all of them now readily available in the U.S. Some of these herbs are effective and inexpensive substitutes for ginseng. Some, when combined with ginseng, will make it more effective. Others, either alone or in formulas, may be better suited to your particular condition than ginseng is. A number of traditional Western herbs may also be used as tonics, although in a different manner than ginseng. I'll explain the properties of all these herbs, describe how they are used in formulas, and tell you where to obtain them.

SELF-MEDICATION WITH CHINESE HERBS

Ginseng and the herbs I describe in this book are widely available in health food stores, herb shops, and Chinese and Korean stores in the U.S. It's my intention with this book to help you take them wisely and effectively. If you're in general good health, there's no reason why you can't take ginseng or formulate your own simple tonic teas or wines. If you're sick, however, especially with an illness of a chronic nature, and you want to take Chinese herbs, you will profit greatly by consulting an acupuncturist or other practitioner of Oriental medicine.

If you're an athlete, and you want to take ginseng or other herbs to improve your performance, I'll explain how to do that too. Even in this case, I hope you'll consider consulting an Oriental medicine practitioner for a formula tailored to your own constitution and sport just as the champion Chinese athletes do.

A naturopathic physician I know, was once asked to define his medicine in one sentence. He thought a moment and replied: "We don't think that petroleum derivatives and the removal of body parts make a good first line of defense against disease." Oriental medicine offers you many alternatives, and indeed excels at restoring balance to your health before you develop a more serious illness. So it's also my hope that this book will be an introduction to the benefits of Oriental medicine, and that you will consider it as an adjunct to conventional medicine. Oriental medicine is often more helpful as a first resort, and as a treatment for chronic illnesses of depletion and exhaustion for which conventional medicine has no effective response.

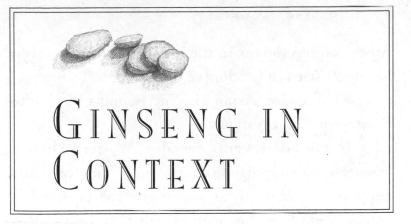

GINSENG IN CONTEXT

There is a well-known tale of four blind men who examined an elephant. One felt the leg, another the trunk, the third the hide, and the last one the tail. They then began to argue about what the elephant was, each on the basis of his own narrow experience of it. The understanding of ginseng in North America today is much like the perceptions of those blind men.

Knowledge of ginseng has come to us from a distant land and from a culture with a very different world-view than our own. Even what we know about American ginseng we learned from the Chinese, who value it highly and have imported thousands of tons of it over the last two-and-a-half centuries. American ginseng was used as a minor remedy by some

American physicians in the nineteenth century, but has never been fully adopted by any Western medical system. Likewise, Asian ginseng remains foreign to Western medical systems.

In the last several decades, Western clinical research has supported the use of ginseng for stress and a few other conditions, and some of its chemical constituents have been identified (I'll discuss this research in Section II). But Western scientific understanding of ginseng is little better than the blind men's understanding of the elephant. We know some things about it, but we still don't know what the whole elephant is.

Ginseng cannot simply be popped like a pill. To really understand how to use it, you will have to understand how the Asians use it. So, in this book, I will take you on a trip into the world of Chinese culture and medicine. I'll introduce you to the reality of *chi* — the basic vital energy. I'll show you how to figure out whether you are "hot," "cold," "excess," "deficient," "exterior," or "interior." All of these are basic concepts in Oriental medicine, and understanding them is essential in order to use ginseng wisely. I'll also introduce you to some other Chinese tonic herbs which may be taken along with ginseng or as substitutes for it.

In short, I'll show you the elephant.

CHAPTER 1

GINSENG IN CHINESE AND AMERICAN HISTORY

"Nobody can imagine that the Chinese and Tartars would set so high a value on this root if it did not constantly provide good effect."

Père Jartoux, *Jesuit Missionary to China, 1711*

"If the people of the United States were educated as to its use, our supply of ginseng would be consumed in our own country and it would be a hard blow to the medical profession."

Dr. Arthur Harding, *ginseng expert, 1909*

Ginseng is the most famous of the Chinese herbs throughout the world, and has been the most valued herb in China since the dawn of written history there. An American variety of ginseng played an important part in the early history and economy of the U.S. after trade in the plant began with China in the 1700s. In this chapter, I'll describe the history of both varieties right up to the present, when they make up one of the fastest-growing categories of herb sales in the U.S.

ASIAN GINSENG

Ginseng has probably been used as a medicine in Asia since the dawn of civilization. Its first written mention was in the first century B.C. in the *Interpretations of Creatures* by You Shi. The earliest mention of ginseng in formal Chinese medical literature appeared in the first century A.D., in the *Shen Nong Ben Cao Jing (The Divine Husbandman's Classic of the Materia Medica)*, the first Chinese book to describe the uses of specific herbs. Ginseng was certainly in use before this in the shamanic medicine that existed for thousands of years before the appearance of the *Classic*. Ginseng probably came into wide use by the Chinese around 3000 B.C., when knowledge of its properties was introduced from Manchuria.

The Divine Husbandman

The authorship of the *Shen Nong Ben Cao Jing* was ascribed to the mythical "Divine Husbandman," the legendary patron of Chinese herbalism who was said to have "tasted the hundred herbs" and given their properties to humanity. He was also said to have introduced agriculture and the breeding of domesticated animals into Chinese culture. The book's actual authorship is unknown.

Chinese herbalism at the time the *Classic* was written was intertwined with the study of alchemy, the goal of which was to achieve longevity. Herbs in the *Classic* were classified according to grade: the lowest grade expels disease; the middle grade corrects imbalances in the body; the highest grade—the one to which ginseng belongs—nourishes life itself. The *Classic* describes ginseng thus:

"It is used for repairing the five viscera, quietening the spirit, curbing the emotion, stopping agitation, removing noxious influence, brightening the eyes, enlightening the mind, and increasing the wisdom. Continuous use leads one to longevity with light weight."

This highest class of drugs comprises the tonic herbs— food-like substances which may be taken for long periods of time with little danger of toxicity. The *Classic* says of them:

"The first class of drugs . . . are considered to perform the work of Sovereigns. They support human life and they resemble heaven. They are not poisonous regardless of the quantity and duration of administration."

The *Classic* described ginseng, but it did not say how to use it in formulas. Around A.D. 200, another Chinese medical text appeared which gave 21 formulas for ginseng out of a total of 113 formulas. By the mid-1600s, 509 out of 2,216 prescriptions in a Korean medical text included ginseng— nearly a fourth of the total.

Man-root

The Chinese name for ginseng, *ren shen*, means "man-root," for its characteristic shape resembling the trunk, arms, and legs of a human being. From the earliest times, the Chinese had stories about ginseng. It was said to have a mystical connection with the constellation Orion, which also has a man shape. One story goes that ginseng was discovered when a woodsman repeatedly heard a voice crying out in the night. Eventually he found the root, shaped like a man, that was making the sound.

Botanical Distinctions

The botanical name for Asian ginseng is *Panax ginseng*. Three other plants in the Panax genus all have tonic properties, but none are identical in their action to Asian ginseng.

Common name: Asian ginseng
Latin name: *Panax ginseng*
Use: Energy tonic, longevity elixir
History: Used from prehistory in China through the present. It is the most renowned herbal tonic in the Chinese culture.

Common name: American ginseng
Latin name: *Panax quinquefolium*
Use: In America, as a general tonic and stimulant. In China, as a mild *chi* tonic, which also moisturizes the system and reduces heat while building strength.
History: Used to some extent by Native American tribes, it was "discovered" in Canada by a Jesuit missionary in 1716; export to China began soon afterward.

Common name: Japanese ginseng
Latin name: *Panax japonicus*
Use: A minor remedy in China, it is used there like American ginseng.

Common name: Tienchi ginseng, sanchi ginseng
Latin name: *Panax pseudoginseng*

Use: To stop bleeding and disperse bruising and swelling after trauma, and for heart disease. Also used as a blood and energy tonic.

History: first appeared in Chinese medical texts around A.D. 1600.

The *Shens*

In Chinese herbalism, which is organized around medicinal action rather than botanical classification, *ren shen* is one of a family of other *shens*—fleshy roots with tonic properties. The *shens* have been sought out and harvested since antiquity in China. The Chinese sometimes refer to any of these as types of ginseng, but they do not generally consider the others as medicinal substitutes for *ren shen*.

TABLE 1.1
THE *SHEN* ROOTS

Chinese Name	Common Name	Uses
ren shen	ginseng	*chi* tonic, especially spleen and lungs
dang shen	codonopsis	spleen and lung tonic
sha shen	adenophora	lung tonic
hsuan shen	scrophularia	kidney tonic
tan shen	salvia	heart tonic
hai er shen	prince ginseng	energy tonic
xi yang shen	American ginseng	yin tonic, for febrile diseases
zhu jie shen	Japanese ginseng	yin tonic, for febrile diseases

Medicinal Uses

Ginseng was, and still is, used in China to increase strength in those who are weak, to build the blood in those who are anemic, to strengthen the appetite, to improve respiration in those short of breath from weakness, to calm the spirit and nerves, as a remedy for impotence, and to increase wisdom in spiritual pursuits. A major use has been to aid in recovery from the low energy and dehydration that follow debilitating feverish diseases. High doses of ginseng are used today in Chinese emergency rooms for patients in critical shock from blood loss or serious chronic disease. I will discuss the Chinese use of ginseng in more detail in Chapter 6.

Asian Ginseng and the West

Tales of ginseng first reached the West via reports from a seventeenth-century Dutch traveler who had been shipwrecked in Korea. Parts of Europe and Russia may have been exposed to ginseng after the Mongol invasions of the thirteenth century. The Mongol soldiers used ginseng to increase their stamina. Ginseng first became known in detail in 1711, through the botanical writings of a Jesuit missionary to Beijing, China, named Père Jartoux. His account was published three years later in English. Jartoux described ginseng this way:

> *"Nobody can imagine that the Chinese and Tartars would set so high a value on this root if it did not constantly provide good effect. Those that are in health often make use of it to render themselves more vigorous and strong; and I am persuaded that it would*

*prove an excellent medicine in the hands of any Euro-
pean who understands pharmacy, if he had but a sufficient quantity of it to make such trials as are
necessary, to examine the nature of it chemically,
and to apply it in a proper quantity according to the
nature of the disease for which it may be beneficial."*

Asian ginseng has never been in great demand in the
West, and medical professionals have paid it little attention.
It was first exported to the U.S. in significant quantity when
Chinese communities began to develop after immigration
during the 1800s. Its use was mainly confined to Chinatowns
until the 1970s, when it became available in health food
stores. It then began to grow in popularity with the public,
mainly based on its reputation as a sexual tonic. With the rise
of the acupuncture profession in this country since the 1970s,
the full medicinal properties of ginseng have become better
known. In 1994, ginseng sales were growing at a rate second only to garlic as an herbal medicine.

AMERICAN GINSENG

A few years after the Jesuit Jartoux published his paper on
Asian ginseng, Joseph Francois Lafitau, a missionary to
Canada, found a North American variety there, now called
American ginseng or *Panax quinquefolium*. Prophetically, Jartoux had said in his original paper, ". . . if it is to be found in
any other country in the world, it may be particularly in
Canada, where the forest and mountains . . . very much
resemble these here [in China]." Lafitau sought out the plant
without success until he described it to some Indians, who
walked a few feet away and brought him one of the roots.

The Chinese, whose own stock of wild indigenous ginseng was becoming rare through over-harvesting, were hungry for export of the new plant and bought it up by the ton. Soon they realized that it had different properties than their own ginseng, but a large trade in it continues even today, when about 95% of the American ginseng crop is exported to China. A half-century before the American Revolution, harvesting ginseng in the wild became a way for trappers, traders, and Indians throughout the Eastern U.S. to obtain ready cash. American ginseng was found throughout the forested areas of the Eastern U.S. and Canada, from Maine through Quebec and Ontario to Wisconsin in the North; to Iowa, Missouri, and Arkansas in the West; and Alabama, Georgia, and South Carolina in the South.

Export of American ginseng has continued unabated now for more than 250 years, and is intimately interwoven with American history. More than 100,000 tons of American ginseng, either harvested in the wild or cultivated on farms, have been exported to China. The demand in Asia is so great that American ginseng now costs about twice as much as Chinese ginseng does in the U.S.

Some Highlights from American History

• The French did a substantial trade in North American ginseng by the early 1700s. This trade prompted them to intrude southward into the lands of the Iroquois, who had a treaty with the British, thus touching off the first skirmishes of century-long conflict between the French and the British in North America.

• Explorer Daniel Boone, who opened up a Southern route for settlers through the Cumberland Gap into Ken-

---

NAMES FOR ASIAN, CHINESE, AND KOREAN GINSENG

Botanical: *Panax ginseng*

The word *Panax* is derived from the Greek words *pan*, which means "all," and *akos*, which means "to cure." *Panax* therefore means "cure all" or "panacea." It received this name in 1843 from the botanist C.A. Meyer, indicating that its "cure-all" properties were well known to European botanists of the time.

Chinese: *ren-shen, jen-seng, schin-seng*

All three names are transliterations of the same original Chinese characters. The two characters are "essence of earth" (or "root") and "in the form of a man."

Japanese: *Ninjin*

Korean: *Insam, yin sam*

NAMES FOR AMERICAN GINSENG

Latin: *Panax quinquefolium* (five-leaved)

Chinese: *xi yang shen.* A literal translation of the Chinese characters is: "root from the Western seas."

Japanese: *Seiyojin*

Korean: *Soyangsam*

Appalachian dialect: *sang, shang*

Mohawk: *Garentoquen* ("thigh and leg of the human body")

Onondaga: *Da-kyen-too-keh*

Oneida: *Ka-lan-da-goo* ("forked plant")

---

tucky and Tennessee, is said to have sold 15 tons of ginseng to a trader in Philadelphia.

    • George Washington noted in his diary that, while traveling west into Ohio, he "met with many mules and packs laden with ginseng going east over the Forbes-Braddock road."

- In 1773, the sloop Hingham left Boston with the most valuable cargo shipped from the colonies to that date: 55 tons of ginseng worth three dollars a pound.
- John Jacob Astor, who amassed one of the greatest early American fortunes through the fur trade, got his first big break exporting ginseng rather than furs. With a partner, he sent a shipload of ginseng to China, bringing back tea. His profits from the excursion were more than $55,000 at a time when a week's pay was only a few dollars. The equivalent today would be about $15,000,000.
- By the late 1800s, the clearing of much of the Eastern forests for agriculture resulted in a greatly reduced natural habitat for ginseng. Cultivation began around 1890.

Native American Uses

From the early 1700s on, ginseng was an important item of trade between Native Americans and the European trappers and traders. Cherokee Indians in North Carolina in the 1800s could obtain the equivalent of two days' pay for a pound of wild ginseng root. Today it is difficult to distinguish which native uses of ginseng were original, and which were learned from the traders who told of the plant's use in China. The following table shows the uses of American ginseng by some tribes:

- Crow: to induce childbirth
- Cherokee: to relieve headaches, muscular cramps, and female problems
- Creek: fresh chewed root applied to wounds to stop bleeding; warm tea for croup in children; hot compress

soaked in ginseng tea for sore throat; ginseng and ginger to sweat out a fever

- Menominee: general tonic to increase physical strength and mental powers
- Ojibwa and Potawatomie: tonic and strengthener of mental powers
- Penobscot: to increase the fertility of women
- Potawatomie: tea of powdered root for sore eyes and earache
- Seneca: a tonic for the elderly
- Sac-Fox: universal remedy; for stomach disorders and menstrual difficulty
- Seminole: to relieve nosebleed and shortness of breath

Ginseng in American Medicine

Although ginseng was used briefly in American medicine during the 1800s, it has never been valued in the U.S. to the extent that it is in Asia. American ginseng was listed as an official medicine in the *U.S. Pharmacopoeia* from 1840 to 1880. American homeopaths used ginseng preparations in tinctures and low potencies in the nineteenth and early twentieth centuries. Eclectic physicians, who specialized in herbal medicine, used ginseng until the 1930s. Its declining use prompted Dr. Arthur Harding, an expert on the medicinal uses of ginseng, to comment in 1909: "If the people of the United States were educated as to its use, our supply of ginseng would be consumed in our own country and it would be a hard blow to the medical profession," because of the improved health of the ginseng consumers. Harding quit his medical practice to devote his full time to cultivating and researching ginseng. He said that ginseng had cured every patient he had used it on where the cause of the illness had been poor nutrition, except for one case of advanced tuber-culosis. In that case, the woman who died said that ginseng had been the only medicine that had done her any good at all.

The 1947 edition of the *United States Dispensatory*, written during the dawning heyday of wonder drugs, includes ginseng in a section devoted to historical curiosities. The authors state: "The extraordinary medicinal virtues formerly attributed to ginseng had no other existence than in the imagination of the Chinese." The text then goes on to say that research had demonstrated that the plant has "a sedative effect and a mildly stimulating action on the vital centers." As we'll see in the following chapters, this mildly stimulating effect is what gives ginseng its power, because mild stimulation over a long period of time can accomplish a restoration of a weakened system that no powerful drug taken for a short time could ever achieve.

CONCLUSION

The demand for American ginseng grew in this country along with the rising popularity of Asian ginseng. Still, only about 5% of the domestic crop, either cultivated or harvested in the wild, remains in the U.S. What are the properties of this mysterious plant, so highly valued in Asia and so much in demand in the U.S.? Conventional medicine, which has never been interested in ginseng, cannot answer this question. To find out, we'll have to take a trip to China.

CHAPTER 2

CHI

To understand in Chinese terms what ginseng does, you will need to learn about *chi* (pronounced "chee"). *Chi* is basic vital energy; there is no parallel concept in modern conventional Western medicine. An understanding of *chi* is so important that you won't be able to use ginseng or other Chinese tonics effectively without it, because ginseng and the tonic herbs build *chi*. And they will work only in the context of a lifestyle and activities that also support and cultivate the *chi*.

A MEDITATION

Step back for a moment from your current beliefs about health, the body, and even the very makeup of the universe. Forget, for the moment, that the universe is made up of atoms, that your body is made up of cells and biochemical processes, and that germs are the cause of disease. Forget the names of any medical conditions you might have or medicines you might be taking for them. You can have these concepts back later. But, for now, sit quietly for a few moments and just experience how you feel. Feel your breath moving in

15

and out in its natural rhythm. Take a few deep breaths. Then meditate and pay attention to the life in yourself. Feel the vibrant life-force in your lungs, your belly, your arms, legs, hands, feet, and head. Feel it animating and vitalizing all your life process: your breathing, your digestion, your muscles, your nervous system, your mind. Feel it throbbing in your heart and moving throughout your circulatory system. Feel it keeping your body warm. Feel and know the *reality* of this life-force.

Now think of someone you know who is in vital good health. This life-force will invariably be strong and radiant in them. You can sense it in a healthy person, and you can almost see it. Think of the vitality radiating from a newborn baby or a young child. Then think of someone you know who is seriously ill with a chronic disease, or who is simply run down. Invariably, this life-force will be dull, their body unanimated, the sparkle gone from their eyes. Think of healthy or sick plants or pets you have had, and remember the vibrant subtle energy around the healthy plant or animal, and the lack of it in the sick one.

Now you are thinking like the Chinese.

CHI AND CHINESE MEDICINE

The reality of this life-force, or *chi*, is the center around which Oriental medicine is built. The atom and the cell are the starting points for the Western view of reality and medicine, but this vital *chi* is the starting point for the traditional Oriental view. It is *chi* that animates everything that lives, grows, and evolves—plants, animals, humans, even atoms and stars—and unites them in one living whole. Western physicists see the universe as composed of matter and energy, and recognize the interaction of the two. Einstein's famous formula $E=mc^2$ states that matter and energy can be transformed into each other in predictable ways. In traditional Oriental philosophy, both matter and energy are expressions of *chi*, and it is *chi* that governs their transformation into each other.

The traditional Chinese physician will acknowledge that we have cells and molecules in our bodies, but will say that it is the *chi* that moves them and makes them alive, and not the other way around. If the *chi* is strong and vibrant, the person will be in good health, be able to withstand stress, accomplish much in life, have a vital sexuality, and be more likely to live a long, natural life. If the *chi* is low and depleted, the person will be tired, run down, and in poor health. If *chi* is completely absent, the person will be dead.

CHI AND ELECTRICITY

An analogy for *chi* is electricity. You can't see electricity, but you can readily see its effects. If you turn on a light switch, the light goes on. If the battery in your flashlight starts to run down, the light grows dim. Electricians and engineers may understand more about electricity than we do, but we have a functional definition of it. We recognize its effects and, because we see them, we acknowledge the existence of electricity without question. In the same way, the Chinese recognize *chi*. They observe its effects in the body, and they don't question its reality any more than we question the reality of electricity. One difference is that electricity flows from an external source — a power station or a battery. *Chi*, on the other hand, resides in the body, interpenetrating it. The body itself is the power source, the battery. And ginseng is for people with a run-down battery.

HERBS, FOODS, LIFESTYLE, AND *CHI*

Just as the Chinese define *chi* by observing it at work, they observe that some plants and animal substances (ginseng and some other tonic herbs and foods) increase the *chi* or help it circulate in the body, improve health, and prolong life. Over the centuries, they did not worry much about exactly *how* it does this or what chemical reactions were involved (although extensive modern research into ginseng and other plants is now conducted in China). They paid more attention to the *way* in which plants affect the *chi*, observing how plant selection, harvesting, preparation and dosage affect the herbal *chi*-building properties.

They have also observed the effects of different life-styles and exercises on the development, maintenance, and circulation of *chi*, and these practices are interwoven with Chinese culture. Go to any public park in China today, and you will see people — sometimes thousands of them at once — practicing *tai chi*, a set of slow-motion, martial-arts-like exercises that build and circulate the *chi* in the body. Even traditional Chinese cooking, with its small, easily digested portions of fresh seafood or freshly butchered meats mixed with stir-fried vegetables, has evolved at least in part because of its *chi*-building properties. I'll discuss the Chinese lifestyle in more detail in Chapter 3, because it is a tenet of Oriental medicine that ginseng and herbs alone will not do the job of building *chi*; they must be taken in the context of a *chi*-building and *chi*-supporting lifestyle.

WHERE *CHI* COMES FROM

The Chinese say that *chi* comes from three sources:

- Prenatal *chi*. This is the *chi* that we are born with, that we receive from our parents at conception. Different individuals may have more or less of it, which at least partly explains why some people naturally have more vitality than others, even at the earliest age. This *chi* resides in the lower abdomen.

- Food *chi*. This *chi* is developed through the digestion of food. Healthy or poor digestion can have an immediate impact on this *chi* and on our overall energy level.

- Air *chi*. The air we breathe is the source of this *chi*. Deep, full breathing and at least light aerobic exercise are necessary in order to have a healthy amount of air *chi*.

HOW *CHI* MOVES

Chi moves and circulates through the body in much the same way that blood does: it moves through channels. Known as *acupuncture meridians* in the West, these channels carry the *chi* from its sources in the digestive system and lungs, and circulate it to every organ and cell in the body. Needles inserted at points along these meridians can affect the flow of *chi* through them. An acupuncturist primarily uses needles on these points to increase or decrease the flow of *chi* to an organ or other part of the body when that flow has become disturbed. Ginseng and tonic herbs, when combined with other herbs in formulas, may also direct the *chi* to specific organs and regions of the body. Like *chi* itself, these meridians are defined functionally. Some may correspond to nerve pathways or blood vessels, and others may have no apparent physical counterpart. But the Chinese have observed their function, and the effects of needles at various points on the flow of *chi*.

Chinese practitioners have also observed that *chi* does not flow evenly through the organs at all times. Each organ has a daily cycle with several hours of peak *chi*, and a natural depression or resting of *chi* at the opposite time of day. The *chi* of the digestive function, for instance, peaks in mid-morning and is at its lowest several hours before midnight. In China, acupuncturists may select a time for treatment — even in the middle of the night — in order to take advantage of this ebb and flow of *chi*.

DISORDERS OF *CHI*

The major disorders of *chi* are *deficiency*, which I will discuss below, and *stagnancy*. *Chi* must be able to flow and circulate throughout the body freely. When it becomes blocked for any reason, disease may result. Imagine a garden hose with water flowing through it. If the hose becomes crimped, the water pressure above the crimp increases and the hose swells there. Below the crimp, the flow is decreased. Similarly, stuck *chi* can result in too much *chi* in one place and not enough in another.

Chinese physicians consider stuck *chi* to be one of the major causes of pain and tension in the areas of the body where *chi* has become stagnant, like the part of the hose above the crimp. Organs or tissues below the site of obstruction may also not function properly due to a local deficiency of *chi*, like the end of the hose with its diminished water flow. Physical or emotional trauma, improper diet, exposure to extremes of weather, lack of exercise, constitutional weak-nesses, or other factors may cause stuck *chi*.

Chi obstruction is very important to consider when taking ginseng or other *chi*-building herbs. To build up the *chi* when it cannot flow freely would be the equivalent of turning up the water pressure in a hose that is crimped. For this rea-son, *chi*-building herbs are not taken when pain, tension, inflammation, emotional frustration, anger, high blood pres-sure, or other signs of *chi* obstruction are present.

WHAT *CHI* DOES

To understand *chi* deficiency—the condition for which gin-seng and tonic herbs are appropriate—let's look at exactly what *chi* does. You'll need to understand how to diagnose deficient *chi* in order to determine whether ginseng is appro-priate for you, or even which variety of it to use.

The functions of *chi* in the human body can be sum-marized as follows:

• *Chi* is responsible for all movement in the body. The involuntary muscles—for example, those in the heart, the arteries, and the intestinal wall—all move because of the presence of *chi*. Likewise, the muscles used in voluntary movement are animated by *chi*. If *chi* is depleted, the breath-ing may be depressed, the digestion sluggish, and the body lethargic with poor endurance and weak lower back, knees, and legs.

• *Chi* supports mental activity. Thinking, remember-ing, planning, learning, and mental growth all rely on *chi*. If *chi* is deficient, the mind may be dull and inefficient.

- *Chi* transmutes food and air into energy and the various substances of the body. If *chi* is deficient, and this transmutation is not effective, the energy will be low and deficiencies may appear in the tissues and substances of the body.

- *Chi* warms the body. With insufficient *chi*, signs of cold may appear, such as a feeling of chilliness, lowered body temperature, or cold hands and feet.

- *Chi* protects the body. A layer of *chi* circulates at the surface of the body between the muscles and the skin. This layer ensures proper functioning of the immune system at the surface of the body, protects the body against external cold and heat, and regulates the sweat glands. If the *chi* is weak, a person may get frequent colds or infections, may feel aversion to cold and wind, and may sweat spontaneously, even without exercising.

- *Chi* holds the organs in place and ensures their proper functioning. If *chi* is seriously deficient, the organs may become prolapsed (they may collapse or fall out of place). Organ function may also be deficient if it is not receiving sufficient *chi*.

Note that not all of the above symptoms are necessarily present when the *chi* is deficient. *Chi* deficiency can affect different functions selectively. A general pattern of the above signs indicates that ginseng or other tonic herbs might be appropriate for you. On the other hand, the opposites of these conditions—overactivity and excitation, feeling of heat rather than cold—would indicate that ginseng is not appropriate for you. I'll give more details about indications and contraindications for ginseng and tonic herbs later in this chapter.

TABLE 2.1
FUNCTIONS OF *CHI* AND SOME POSSIBLE SIGNS OF ITS DEFICIENCY

Movement of voluntary and involuntary muscles	Depressed breathing, quiet voice, poor digestion, heart palpitations or racing heart, physical weakness and fatigue, lack of endurance, weak back and legs
Thinking, reasoning, learning, remembering	Dull and lethargic mind, poor memory
Transmutation of food and air into the substances and energy of the body	Low energy, malnutrition, low metabolism, depressed sexual function, menstrual irregularities
Maintenance of body warmth	Depressed body temperature, general feeling of cold, cold hands and feet
Protection of the body from heat, cold, and infection	Frequent colds, aversion to wind, spontaneous sweating
Stabilization of the organs within the body	Prolapsed organs
Organ functioning	Dysfunction of any organ in the body

CHI AND BLOOD

In Oriental medicine, *chi* and blood are intimately connected. The blood arises from the mixing of *chi* derived from food and *chi* derived from air. So blood is dependent on *chi*. Circulating blood then nourishes the entire body. But throughout the process, *chi* and blood remain inseparable, almost like two sides of a piece of paper. The *chi* of the heart pumps the blood, and the *chi* of other organs and vessels contains the blood and maintains blood pressure. So the Chinese say that "*chi* is the commander of the blood." But *chi* is also dependent on blood, because the tissues require adequate nutrition for *chi* to function in them. So the Chinese also say that "blood is the mother of *chi*."

We'll see in Chapter 12 that some tonic herbs, such as ginseng, are primarily *chi* tonics. Others are primarily blood tonics. Because of the interdependence of *chi* and blood, a deficiency of one is often accompanied by a deficiency of the other, and *chi* and blood tonics are often combined in formulas. Many people in China take ginseng by itself. But in formal Oriental medicine, it is almost always combined with other tonics, usually blood tonics. The list below shows some of the symptoms of blood deficiency. Ginseng and other *chi* tonics are often used in China to treat anemia, the Western term for some of the symptoms of blood deficiency.

Some symptoms of blood deficiency:
    pale complexion
    dizziness
    spots before the eyes
    pale tongue
    pale lips
    pale nails
    insomnia
    palpitations
    poor memory
    poor appetite
    mental fatigue
    menstrual irregularity
    emaciation

VITAL ENERGY IN THE HISTORY OF WESTERN MEDICINE

The central role of a vital energy in health and disease is not a completely foreign concept in the history of Western medicine, but it has been lost in modern conventional medicine. Harris Coulter, in his book *Divided Legacy*, traces both "vitalist" and "materialist" medicine back to the roots of European history. He concludes that these two approaches ebbed and flowed like tides throughout Western history. We are probably past a high tide of conventional materialistic medicine now, as alternative, vitalist systems of medicine are enjoying an upsurge in popularity and even attracting the attention of conventional physicians.

The Western concept of vital force is not as well developed as the Chinese concept of *chi*. Vital force, as seen in the West, is a vague but important energy that animates the body, coordinates bodily functions, and produces symptoms in an attempt to heal any imbalance. Western vitalist systems include homeopathy, naturopathy, chiropractic, and medical herbalism. The essential aims of these vitalist systems are to create a context in the lifestyle that supports the vital force, to use medicines or methods that help it to express itself in the body, to remove obstructions to its harmonious expression, and to never suppress symptoms that the vital force produces in attempts to heal the body. Conventional medicine, on the other hand, systematically suppresses symptoms as they arise, usually at the expense of a patient's overall vitality.

Until about 300 years ago, most of Western medicine was vitalist. Even a hundred years ago, homeopathy had a strong position and a large following in the U.S. Let's look briefly at some of these vitalist systems that are increasingly popular in the U.S.:

Homeopathy

Homeopathic doctors use highly diluted substances, that have no direct physiological effect, in order to influence the vitality of the patient. With increased vitality, the patient's own body and unconscious intelligence can throw off the disease from within.

Naturopathic Medicine

Practitioners in this profession employ diet, exercise, medical herbalism, spinal manipulation, hydrotherapy, homeopathy, some principles of Chinese medicine, and other methods to enhance the vital force and restore its activity in the body.

Chiropractic

Chiropractors adjust misalignments of the spine that impinge on the functioning of the nerves passing through the spine. This is a vitalist system, because it is essentially the flow of vital force that is blocked. Some chiropractors may be overly dogmatic about the spinal misalignments being the sole cause of disease. But whether you call it nerve force that is blocked in the spine, or see it as *chi* blocked in the meridians along the spine, or even say that the soft tissues around the misalignment block the flow, many millions of people have experienced healing and increased vitality following a course of spinal manipulation.

Medical Herbalism

Some medical herbalists use herbs the same way that conventional physicians do. They will give "this" herb for "that" condition without looking at the overall picture of the patient. Other herbalists, however, use a vitalist approach, and select their herbs and other methods to support the vital force in the body.

Oriental Medicine

Acupuncture and Chinese herbalism are spreading rapidly in the U.S., with at least 22 schools of Oriental medicine now turning out licensed acupuncturists and herbalists.

Ayurvedic Medicine

This medicine from India, like Chinese medicine, relies primarily on diet, herbs, and exercises (yoga) to restore balance in the body and support the vital force.

An Advantage of Vitalist and Tonic Medicine

I have a friend—a naturopathic physician and acupuncturist—who used to work in an AIDS clinic in San Francisco that was run by conventional medical doctors. One of the M.D.s once said to her, "You know what I like best about your kind of medicine? You can treat people when there's nothing wrong with them!" He meant that with her methods, which treated disorders of *chi* and blood, she could help patients who did not have a disease that fit into a conventional diagnostic category.

This is the great strength of Chinese medicine and other vitalist systems. It's also the great strength of ginseng and tonic herbs. About half the people visiting a regular M.D. leave the office without a diagnosis, because there's not yet anything "wrong with them." They feel run down, sick, tired, or anxious, but nothing objectively abnormal shows up in their blood tests or physical examination. They are actually in the first stage of chronic disease, but nothing has become noticeably deranged in their bodies yet. Sometimes an M.D. will give such a patient an antidepressant or a sedative drug, or refer them to a psychiatrist saying, "it's all in your head." Such a patient would surely receive a prompt and detailed diagnosis from a Chinese practitioner, and receive treatment—often with tonic herbs—based on that diagnosis.

A comparison of the Western and the Chinese view of a patient with the "blahs" is like the difference between English-speakers and the Eskimos in their view of snow. English-speaking North Americans have only one word for snow because they do not require more than that to function in their environment. Eskimos, on the other hand, have more than 30 different words for snow, all necessary for survival in a snowy environment. Conventional medicine has no language for the indefinable state of feeling bad without a diagnosable disease. Chinese doctors, however, have a wide vocabulary for these states; their terms are just as important to their medical system as is the differentiation of types of snow to the Eskimo.

This well-developed analysis of "pre-illness" states arises from the goal of traditional Chinese medicine: to treat disharmonies *before* they become serious diseases. An ancient Chinese text says: "To treat disease after it has already arisen is like digging a well when you are already thirsty, or forging swords after war has already broken out." Oriental medicine can certainly treat the whole range of advanced illnesses as well, but it is early-stage harmonizing and tonic therapy that sets it apart from conventional Western medicine.

MY STORY

In one recent year, I was under tremendous stress. I had lost a major publishing contract which accounted for more than half of my income. My fiancée got cold feet and backed out of plans for marriage. I was also unemployed for three months. Eventually, I got a book contract with a very short deadline. As a result, I had to write into the night, sometimes until dawn, five or six nights a week for about six weeks, even as my bills mounted and remained unpaid. I was in my late forties, and I did not have the stamina for these all-nighters that I had when I was younger. Despite this invitation to exhaustion, I continued to exercise vigorously, doing up to 10 hours a week of aerobic exercise to "let off steam."

By the time I finished writing the book, I was in a state of physical collapse. I developed insomnia so severe that, even when I slept, I could not get into deep sleep. My adrenal glands were in a "fight-or-flight" state 24 hours a day. What's more, my feet swelled up so severely that, for a few days, I couldn't get my shoes on. For about three weeks, I was too mentally exhausted to sit and write for even five minutes. The swelling lessened somewhat, but it persisted for weeks.

The swelling was of the sort that, if you poked your finger into it, an indentation would remain for a long time afterward—"pitting edema," in conventional medicine. This kind of edema is usually considered the sign of grave disease. Heart failure, kidney failure, liver failure, or terminal cancer are some of the possibilities, and I accepted the fact that I might not have long to live. I sought out the best conventional medical specialists I could find, including an ultrasound specialist who had written a book on the subject. The first doctor I saw was so alarmed by my symptoms that he considered sending me to the emergency room. After extensive medical testing, the doctors ruled out all the usual causes of such symptoms. My heart, lungs, liver, and kidneys were unusually healthy, and an ultrasound examination showed no tumors. The last doctor I saw, a specialist in internal medicine who was open to alternative medicine, said that my condition was a mystery, and gave me "permission" to try alternative methods.

My symptoms would have been no mystery to a Chinese practitioner. In Chinese medicine, the "Kidney" (a translation from Chinese medicine that does not correspond exactly to the physical kidneys) is responsible for water balance in the body. This Chinese "Kidney" includes the physical kidney function, but it also involves the glands and hormones that handle water balance, stress reactions, and the sexual function. Three things that tend to deplete this Kidney function are: excess stress, staying up too late at night, and over-exercise, all of which I had engaged in. My actual Chinese diagnosis was beyond the scope of this book, but, in short, I had severely deficient *chi* which had deranged the ability of my Kidney to maintain water balance.

I treated the condition at first by using four vitalist systems of medicine: naturopathic medicine, hydrotherapy, chiropractic, and homeopathy. I moderated my exercise, took several week-long vacations, and increased my daily meditation routine. After about three months, the edema was gone. I had mostly recovered, but my energy remained somewhat low. I felt that I was running on four spark plugs with a six-cylinder engine. Eventually, I took a course of American ginseng and some of the other tonic herbs that I'll discuss in Chapter 13. Within two weeks, I was restored to full vitality—more than I had felt in years. Ever since, I make sure I take a short course of tonic herbs whenever I am under unusual stress or have to stay up late at night.

The main point of my story is that, although I was sicker than I have ever been in my life, I had absolutely no diagnosable Western condition. There was "nothing wrong with me." This is because conventional medicine does not recognize the vital force, or the *chi*, and has no methods for building it up. Even the other natural methods I was using could only take me so far.

At the beginning of this chapter, I asked you to set aside your beliefs about conventional medicine. I hope you have now learned something about *chi*, but I won't ask you to abandon Western medicine completely. I have nothing against conventional medicine, and use it as I judge it to be appropriate. I am alive today because of a round of antibiotics that I took for a serious systemic infection as a young adult. I would be blind in one eye today had I not had eye surgery as a child. And I have friends who are alive because of heroic organ transplants. But for many people, a vitality-centered approach, including ginseng and tonic herbs when appropriate, is the best first line of defense against disease; at the very least, it is a valuable complement to conventional Western treatments. Even people with a diagnosable conventional disease may have underlying *chi* and blood deficiencies as the cause of their ailment. As one ancient Chinese text says: "If blood and *chi* fall into disharmony, a hundred diseases may arise."

Another point of my story is that I took the ginseng and tonic herbs in the context of important *chi*-cultivating lifestyle changes: rest, recreation, moderation of excess exercise, meditation, and other vitalist medical treatments. This brings us to the next chapter, in which I'll discuss some *chi*-building practices from Chinese culture and suggest ways in which you can maintain and develop your own *chi*.

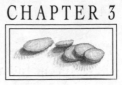

CHAPTER 3

A CHI-CULTIVATING LIFESTYLE

I once had an experience that dramatically demonstrated for me how Chinese treatments are always seen in the context of lifestyle. I consulted an expert Chinese herbalist and acupuncturist who had recently moved to the U.S. after being in charge of a hospital ward in Beijing for more than 20 years. She was preparing for her Oregon acupuncture board exams and studying the English required for medical interviews. For practice, I let her interview me and take my case. I considered myself lucky because she had both a traditional Oriental Medical Doctor degree and a conventional M.D. degree, and was recognized as an expert in her profession in China.

My chief symptoms were a chronic mild cough and insomnia. No doubt, an American M.D. would have given me a cough syrup and a sedative and sent me on my way.

This doctor asked me a few questions, analyzed my pulse (in six different locations along the wrist), and looked at my tongue. After less than two minutes of examination, she said, "You have deficient Lung *chi*," which is a diagnosis typical of chronic cough with shortness of breath. Then she said, "You also have deficient *chi*." She further stated that the deficient *chi* was not new, but was itself chronic. Then she surprised me by saying, "I could give you herbs and acupuncture, but they won't do any good unless you change the way you think." She said that I worried too much, and as a result worked too hard, which caused the deficiency. She said that she could also give me herbs to make me sleep, but that it was the mental worry that was keeping me awake.

This approach is typical of a Chinese practitioner. The acupuncturist's needles and herbs are viewed as allies in restoring harmony to the body, but the traditional Chinese practitioner would never expect them to do the job by themselves. China has a culture that is conscious of *chi*—what depletes it and what builds it—and Chinese medicine must be understood in the context of this cultural viewpoint. The Chinese take ginseng and other tonic herbs in addition to a *chi*-preserving, *chi*-cultivating lifestyle. Of course, it would be a mistake to overgeneralize the cultural practices of a country that accounts for about one-fifth of the world's population; there is certainly a wide variety of behavior among its people. However, the following are some elements of the Chinese culture that help build and preserve *chi*.

FOOD

Most Americans have a general concept of the Chinese diet based on eating in Chinese restaurants. The meals are simple: rice, stir-fried dishes, soups, egg rolls, and so on. Meats and

seafood may be included in the stir-fries, but in modest quantities. Compared to an American meal of steak, potatoes, and
a vegetable, a Chinese meal is lower in fat, lighter, and much
easier to digest.

We saw in the last chapter that digested food is the
most important source of *chi*. A friend of mine who travels
regularly to China says that the Chinese "eat their *chi*." The
vegetables that the Chinese eat are more likely to be locally
grown and fresh, still vibrant with their own *chi*. Freezing
and canning of vegetables depletes their vitality. Meats and
seafood in China are also more likely to be fresh and recently
slaughtered or caught.

The American habit of eating large meals of hard-to-
digest and depleted foods, and gulping junk food (an average
of one-third of a pound per person a day), leads to digestive
disorders and malabsorption of food. This tends to deplete
the *chi*-building properties of the digestive system. In my
practice as an herbalist, I have often seen people regain their
energy simply by changing their diet and correcting digestive
disorders with herbal medicines.

The Chinese are also more likely to eat earlier in the
day, when the food can be digested and transformed into *chi*
when it is most needed. Many Americans skip breakfast or
eat lightly, then have their main meal at dinner when it is
harder to digest and when the energy demands of the day
are already over. I'll explain this principle in greater detail in
Chapter 5 on the Chinese Organ Systems.

EXERCISE

Most Chinese people lead more active lives than do Americans. Scenes from Chinese cities show the streets crowded
with bicycles and pedestrians. Manual labor on farms or in

cities is much more common than in America. Americans are more likely to ride in cars, to work at desk jobs, or to sit in front of a television than are the Chinese. Regular, moderate exercise increases respiration, circulates *chi* and blood, and stimulates digestion. When Americans exercise, it tends to be sporadic—a few times a week rather than every day—and heavily aerobic. Heavy exercise can deplete the *chi* rather than build it.

REST

The Chinese sleep an average of eight to nine hours a night, and sometimes even longer during the winter months in agricultural regions. This helps to restore the *chi*. Americans, on the other hand, sleep an average of seven-and-a-half hours a night, and a third of Americans sleep six hours a night or less. Ginseng and the tonic herbs can build energy, but probably won't overcome the *chi*-depletion caused by insufficient rest.

CHI-BUILDING EXERCISES

Millions of Chinese practice the graceful, slow-motion, martial-arts-like exercise, known as *tai chi*, which helps to build and circulate the *chi*. Another type of exercise performed in China is *chi gong*. These vigorous yoga-like breathing exercises and movements are often prescribed medically to build the *chi* or to circulate it through the meridians. Americans have no equivalent to these exercises.

MODERATION OF SEXUAL INDULGENCE

Here we are entering an area that is sure to be foreign to most Americans. In Western culture and in modern medicine, we have no concept of the connection between sex and health, except for the possibility of contracting a sexually transmitted disease. But traditional healing systems around the world, including traditional Chinese medicine, Ayurvedic medicine, and Arabic medicine, all emphasize the importance of conserving sexual energy. They see the consequences of overindulgence as including impotence, premature ejaculation, lower back pain, weakness in the legs, dizziness, poor memory, spiritual malaise, and general low energy. Even in the West, medical-level herbal texts from a hundred years ago list so many remedies for "ill effects of excess sexual indulgence" that it is clear that treatment of this condition was considered a routine part of office practice. Likewise, the older homeopathic texts list many remedies for such overindulgence.

In Ayurveda, it is sometimes said that more than four ejaculations in a month will lead to a decline in the mental or physical faculties of males. In Arabic medicine, one text suggests that more than three ejaculations in a month may lead to the same result, although different people will have different capacities. The Chinese are less specific, noting that frequency of sex without ill consequences can vary widely with the individual, the season, and other factors in the lifestyle. But Chinese medical practitioners routinely diagnose and treat syndromes associated with overindulgence. The usual treatment is to recommend moderation, while at the same time prescribing herbal formulas to build sexual stamina. Women are less likely to lose energy in the sexual act, but may develop the same kind of syndromes after childbirth, especially after having many children.

Taiwanese traditional practitioners have prescriptions for sexual abstinence to accompany many of their treatments. I once overheard an acupuncturist from Taiwan telling a

TABLE 3.1
SOME DIFFERENCES BETWEEN THE
CHINESE AND AMERICAN LIFESTYLES

Chinese Culture	American Culture
underfed	overfed
simple food	complicated food
deficiency through malnutrition	deficiency through poor quality food and malabsorption
active	sedentary
thin	obese
exposed to elements of weather	sheltered from extremes of weather
engage in *chi*-building exercises	more likely to overexercise
sexual moderation	sexual overindulgence

Some things that deplete *chi*:	Some things that build *chi*:
Poor quality of food: sugars, junk food, ice cream, pizza, etc.	appropriate diet (simple, high-quality foods)
digestive malabsorption	healthy digestive system
sedentary lifestyle	mild-to-moderate exercise
overactivity	proper sleep
overwork	rest and recreation
excess weight	sexual moderation
overexercise	meditation *tai chi, chi gong*, yoga
insufficient sleep	
stimulant abuse	
overindulgence in sex	

woman that he could help her avoid surgery for torn shoulder ligaments if she would take acupuncture treatments and herbs, and refrain from having sex for two months.

The idea of sexual moderation as a health-protecting practice is well-known throughout the Chinese culture. Taoist practitioners, who probably first formulated the concept of *chi* and observed the meridians and organ systems during their meditations, have advocated this for thousands of years. These monks, unlike Western celibate monks, were usually married, and observed the intimate connection between their sexual activity and their mental and spiritual progress. They also developed sexual practices that prevented ejaculation by the male. Stories of Chinese emperors using these practices appear throughout Chinese history. Books on Taoist sexual practices are available in English in many bookstores in the U.S.

These beliefs are not isolated to a few eccentric monks or esoteric medical practitioners, but are widely known, recognized, and practiced in the Chinese culture. In the 1980s, the Chinese government published and widely disseminated a brochure about sexuality. This was newsworthy here in the West because the Chinese society is somewhat puritanical, and open discussion of sex by a government agency raised eyebrows among the Western journalists. The government considered it a public health matter. Besides education about sexually transmitted disease, one of the injunctions was against excessive sex. The pamphlet said that "excessive" might be a very different frequency for different individuals, but that the first sign of overindulgence would be fatigue after sex.

Many Americans seek out ginseng when they hear that it will enhance sexual performance. Ginseng can help to restore a system that has been depleted through overindulgence, although several other tonic herbs — *he shou wu* and dendrobium, for example — are better for this purpose. A Chinese-style program of deliberate moderation accompanied by tonic herbal treatments might be more effective in building a satisfying sexual life than simply overstimulating the system to unnatural heights. According to the Chinese, restraint—not outright denial—can enhance health, vigor, memory, creativity, and spiritual happiness.

Table 3.1 compares some of the lifestyle differences between the Chinese and Americans and lists some habits that either deplete or build the *chi*. If you have deficient *chi*, and are thinking of taking ginseng or other tonic herbs, you will be more successful in your recovery if you make some changes in your lifestyle.

CHAPTER 4

GINSENG AND CONSTITUTIONAL MEDICINE

To continue our journey into the Chinese medical world view, I'll now explain constitutional medicine and how ginseng use fits into it. A person's constitution is much like the constitution of a nation: the basic rules by which a country makes its laws and runs its affairs. Different nations have different ground rules, and so do different individuals. No two individuals have an identical constitution, but they fall into certain categories of Chinese medicine. One individual is naturally robust, another frail. One is hot-blooded, and another always has cold hands and feet. One thrives in dry mountain air, and another feels best by the ocean. One puts on weight with the slightest dietary indiscretion, and another cannot put on weight no matter what they eat. Western medicine ignores such considerations, but they are perhaps the most important considerations in Chinese medicine.

Western medicine looks at diseases rather than at individuals. Any of the types above might have arthritis, or an ulcer, or high blood pressure, and conventional medicine will treat each disease in the same way regardless of the patient's constitution. Chinese medicine, on the other hand, takes the symptoms of the disease into account, but will select treatment on the basis of the patient's constitution. To understand the significance of this, let's meet two fictional characters.

The Businessman and the Grandmother

Standing before us are a businessman and a grandmother. Each has an ulcer. The businessman is angry, red-faced, robust, overweight, aggressive, and hard-driving, with a pulse pounding so hard that you can almost see it beating in his temples. He is hot, he kicks off the covers at night, and he likes cold drinks. The grandmother is frail and thin. Her face is pale, her voice soft. She is weak and tired. Her pulse is so thin that you can barely find it. She has cold hands and feet, wears extra layers of clothes, and likes warm drinks. She is more fearful than angry.

Although both of these patients have ulcers, they have very different constitutions. A practitioner of Western medicine would probably give each of them a drug to reduce the secretion of stomach acid. A practitioner of Chinese medicine, however, would give them entirely different diagnoses, and treat them differently.

The businessman would receive herbs, diet, acupuncture, or exercises to reduce the stress and the heat in his system. He might receive herbs with a bitter flavor to "cool" his digestive tract. The grandmother would receive treatments to warm her up and increase her strength. She might receive warming herbs such as ginger, or sweet ones such as licorice, for her digestive problems. Most important, she would be treated with tonic therapy, possibly with ginseng, while the businessman would not. In fact, tonic therapy could make the businessman's symptoms worse. In the U.S., where the public is generally unaware of the appropriate use of ginseng, the aggressive businessman would be more likely to use it to enhance his drive, while the grandmother, who could really benefit from it, would probably be unaware that it exists.

SIX PRINCIPLES

Chinese medicine uses three basic polarities to assess the state of a patient. Bear in mind that almost no patient is purely of one type, but will usually fall toward one end of a spectrum on the polarities of "excess vs. deficiency," "hot vs. cold," and "exterior vs. interior." The Chinese also have another five-phase method of constitutional evaluation, but the six principles above will suffice for the purposes of understanding how to take ginseng and the tonic herbs. These herbs are used in China for cold, deficiency, and interior patterns, and are avoided or used with caution in hot, excess, and exterior conditions. The hundreds of millions of ginseng consumers in China understand these distinctions well. By learning them, American ginseng users can avoid the Ginseng Abuse Syndrome, which I discuss in detail in Chapter 7. See the accompanying checklists to determine where you fall on these polarities. Note that people may have some signs on both sides of the polarity, but usually they will have a preponderance on one or the other.

TABLE 4.1
CHECKLIST FOR EXCESS AND DEFICIENCY

Excess (The Businessman)		Deficiency (The Grandmother)	
Agitation	___	Lethargy	___
Active limbs	___	Curled posture	___
Desire for activity	___	Desire for quiet	___
Red or flushed complexion	___	White or pale complexion	___
Loud voice	___	Low voice	___
Restless and talkative	___	Little desire to speak	___
Rough breathing	___	Shortness of breath	___
Distended abdomen	___	Soft abdomen, or distention with intermittent relief	___
Complaint worse with pressure	___	Complaint better with pressure	___
Complaint better with activity	___	Complaint better with rest	___
Strong pulse	___	Weak pulse	___
Wide pulse	___	Narrow pulse	___
Thick tongue coat	___	Little or no tongue coat	___

Excess vs. Deficiency

The most important guide for the use of ginseng and
other tonic herbs is the "excess vs. deficiency" polarity. Note
that "deficiency" as a Chinese term may have no relation to
"deficiency" in Western medicine, such as "calcium deficiency." The Chinese term is sometimes translated as "vacu-
ity" or "emptiness." In our example above, the businessman
had an excess constitution, and the grandmother a deficient
one. Ginseng and tonics are contraindicated in excess conditions, which might be worsened by taking these herbs.

Ginseng and other tonics, on the other hand, are the ideal treatment for deficiency patterns. In Chapter 12, I'll go into much greater detail on how to evaluate deficiency.

One kind of deficiency pattern that requires caution in using tonics, especially Chinese ginseng, is deficiency with heat signs. Chinese ginseng is contraindicated in patterns which include heat signs.

Hot vs. Cold

The hot patient does not necessary run a fever, but you can take one look and see the heat. They usually feel hot subjectively, even if their temperature is 98.6°. They may have a

TABLE 4.2
CHECKLIST FOR HOT AND COLD

Hot		Cold	
Red complexion	___	Pale or white complexion	___
Aversion to heat	___	Aversion to cold	___
Agitation	___	Cold hands and feet	___
Fewer layers of clothing, bedding	___	Extra layers of clothing, bedding	___
Thirst	___	No thirst	___
Desire for warm drinks	___	Desire for cold drinks	___
Scanty urination	___	Plentiful urine	___
Dark-colored urine	___	Clear urine	___
Hard stool	___	Thin stool	___
Diarrhea with foul-smelling stool	___	Light-colored stool	___
Red tongue	___	Pale tongue	___
Yellow coat on tongue	___	No coat or white coat on tongue	___
Rapid pulse	___	Deep pulse and/or slow pulse	___

TABLE 4.3
CHECKLIST FOR EXTERIOR AND INTERIOR

Exterior	Interior
Symptoms are located in external organs (skin, muscles, joints, mucous membranes, lungs)	Symptoms are located in the internal organs (the digestive tract, heart, kidneys, bladder, uterus, etc.)
pulse floating near the surface of the skin ___	pulse deep toward the wrist bones
fever ___	
headache ___	
aversion to cold ___	
aversion to wind ___	
pain in the muscles ___	
pain in the joints ___	
nasal congestion ___	
cough ___	
thin, white tongue coat ___	

red face; they may be agitated and restless; their pulse will usually be fast. Cold patients may likewise have a normal body temperature, but they will feel cold. They will be pale, and their pulse will be slow. Asian ginseng and other warming tonics are not appropriate for self-medication in deficient patients with heat signs. American ginseng, on the other hand, is ideal for the hot and deficient patient. I'll explain the differentiation between these two ginsengs later in this section. Tonic herbs are classified as heating or cooling, and are selected for a particular patient on the basis of signs of cold or heat, respectively.

Exterior vs. Interior

The terms "exterior" and "interior" refer to the area of the body where symptoms are predominant. Exterior pat-

TABLE 4.4
THE PULSE AND TONGUE IN THE SIX CATEGORIES

	Hot	Cold	Excess	Deficient	Exterior	Interior
Pulse		slow	wide, firm	narrow, weak	at the surface	deep
Tongue		pale				
Tongue		white	thick	no coat or thin coat		

terns have a concentration of symptoms at the surface of the body: the skin, muscles, and mucous membranes. Most common acute illnesses, such as colds or flu, allergies, muscle and joint aches, headaches, and skin rashes, are exterior. Other complaints without such external manifestations are considered to be interior. Ginseng and other tonics are contraindicated in all exterior conditions, which the herbs may aggravate. This means that if you are taking ginseng and you catch a cold, you should stop taking the ginseng until the acute condition passes. Exterior and interior patterns may also be characterized by heat or cold, but for the purposes of this book, be aware that pronounced surface symptoms usually contraindicate ginseng and other tonic herbs. Also note that if you have an illness, you should consult a physician, whether Western or Chinese, rather than attempting to self-medicate with tonic herbs. In Appendix B, I list places where you can locate an acupuncturist or other natural physician.

CONCLUSION

If you have checked your own constitution and symptoms against the lists in this chapter, you have laid the groundwork for determining whether ginseng is appropriate for you, which kind to take, and what other tonic herbs or formulas are best for you. If you learn nothing else from this chapter, remember this: tonics are for deficient constitutions. They may be used in special circumstances to improve performance, by athletes, for example, because athletes have a deficient constitution relative to the level of their activity. They might be used cautiously by normally healthy people who are under stress. I'll cover the use of tonic herbs by athletes in Chapter 16. Athletes will generally do better to take a balanced tonic formula, the way Chinese athletes do, rather than to simply take ginseng.

CHAPTER 5

THE CHINESE ORGAN SYSTEMS

At the beginning of this section, I told the story of the blind men and the elephant. Here we come to another major feature of the "elephant": the Chinese organ systems. You will need to have some knowledge of these systems in order to understand what ginseng and the other Chinese tonic herbs do. Ginseng's remarkable medicinal action, from the Chinese point of view, is that to some extent it can benefit all the organ systems, while most tonics only benefit a few.

ORGANS EAST AND WEST

The names of the Chinese organ systems can be confusing, because, when translated, they have the same names as Western physical organs. Chinese medicine, which evolved in a culture that discouraged cutting open the physical body, defines functional systems and relationships that often have no apparent connection to each other from the Western point of view. The Chinese Heart (*xin*), for instance, includes the physical heart, the propulsion of blood throughout the body, the tongue, the complexion of the face, and the conscious mind. Herbal or acupuncture treatments for this Heart system might benefit physical heart disease, or might just as readily be given for forgetfulness, excessive dreaming, or insomnia—disorders of the consciousness. The Chinese might not say that the physical heart has a direct cause-and-effect relationship with the conscious mind, yet even in the West, we recognize that a shock to the conscious mind can affect the heart.

Just as the Chinese developed a functional definition of *chi* (remember our example of electricity and the light switch), over many centuries they observed functional relationships in the body and psyche that they defined as organ systems. In my opinion, it would be better to keep the original Chinese terms, as we do with *chi*, than to mix the languages of the two systems in this confusing way. These translations are now a standard convention in Oriental medicine in the West, however, so I'll use them throughout the book. To make things clearer, I will capitalize the Chinese term, while keeping it lowercase when it is used in the Western context.

ORGAN *CHI*

In Chapter 2, I mentioned that one of the types of *chi* supplies vitality and enables the function of each organ system. An overall *chi* deficiency may manifest itself primarily in one or several organs, and the tonic herbs I'll cover in Chapter 13 are selected accordingly. Ginseng, or one of its substitutes, is invariably prescribed by Chinese physicians in formulas to treat deficient organ function when there is an overall *chi* deficiency. If you have a physical disease, or any serious disorder, you should probably not self-medicate with these herbs. If you want Chinese herbal treatment, I've provided a referral number in Appendix B where you can locate a trained practitioner of Chinese medicine.

Imbalances of *chi* in the organs can be complex. For instance, if *chi* is not flowing properly, it may be deficient in one organ system, but in excess in another. In this case, if you took ginseng or tonics, you might help the deficient organ, but you might also increase the excess in the other, increasing your discomfort. A trained acupuncturist can ensure that the *chi* of the organs is properly balanced, and can recommend tonic formulas tailored to your particular body type and condition.

THE FIVE VISCERA

The Divine Husbandman's Classic, the oldest book of Chinese herbal medicine, says that Asian ginseng is used for "repairing the 5 viscera." Although Oriental medicine recognizes 12 organ systems, 5 are considered the most important: the Spleen, the Lung, the Liver, the Heart, and the Kidney. Table 5.1 gives a brief overview of each of the 12 systems. I'll describe the 5 major ones in more detail, and show how Asian ginseng affects them. Remember that the Chinese concept of an organ system includes far more than the physical organ. Each of the Chinese organ systems has a pattern of influence that affects the entire body in one way or another.

The Spleen

In order to understand how the Chinese use ginseng and other *chi* tonics, the Spleen is the most important organ to learn. The Spleen is like the Grand Central Station of *chi*.

TABLE 5.1
THE CHINESE ORGAN SYSTEMS

Bladder (*pang-quang*)
The *pang-quang* receives and excretes the urine.

Gall Bladder (*∂an*)
The *∂an* includes the function of the physical gallbladder, and the
mental function of decision-making.

Heart (*xin*)
Xin includes the physical heart and its function, the propulsion of
blood, the arterial system, the complexion, the tongue, the external
ear, the conscious mind, and the containment of the spirit.

Kidney (*∫hen*)
The *∫hen* includes the physical kidneys, the adrenal glands, ovaries,
testes, brain, spinal column, bones, teeth, anus, urethra, and inner
ear, and the functions of stress-response, fluid balance, reproduction,
and growth. The Kidney assists in respiration.

Large intestine (*∂a-chang*)
The *∂a-chang* includes the physical large intestine and the function of
the elimination of solid wastes and psychological release.

Liver (*gan*)
The *gan* includes the physical liver, the tendons, ligaments, and external genitalia, and the functions of storing blood and regulating the
smooth and orderly flow of blood and emotions.

Lung (*fei*)
The *fei* includes the physical lungs and their functions, the skin, the
hair, the refinement of *chi*, the maintenance of rhythm in the body,
the immune defenses at the surface of the body, and psychological
boundaries.

The organ *chi* of the Spleen—"Spleen *chi*"—is like the power
supply of the Spleen itself. It drives Spleen functions that
have far-reaching effects in the body. The Spleen *chi* trans-
forms food into *chi* and blood. It sends this transmuted food

TABLE 5.1 *continued*

Pericardium (*xin-bao*)
The function of the *xin-bao* is to protect the heart. This organ was described in the Chinese classics, but today the functions are held to come under the Heart.

Spleen (*pi*)
The *pi* includes the physical spleen, pancreas, lymph network, large muscles, flesh, lips, and eyelids, and the function of extracting and converting nutrients into blood and *chi*, nourishing the muscles, and keeping the blood in its proper channels.

Stomach (*wei*)
The *wei* prepares the food for digestion, and its downward-moving *chi* sends it to the Spleen.

Small Intestine (*xiao-chang*)
The *xiao-chang* includes the upper intestinal tract below the stomach and liver, and the function of separating out the useful components of food and transmitting wastes to the organs of elimination.

Triple Burner (*san jiao*)
The *san jiao* has no corresponding organ in Western medicine. The "upper burner" is the area of the body above the diaphragm, including the head; the "middle burner" is the area of the body below the diaphragm but above the navel; the lower burner is the area of the body below the navel. The Triple Burner is the functional relationship between all these organs that regulate water balance.

---

essence up to the lungs, where *chi* from the air is added to it and blood is formed. Spleen *chi* also transports the generated *chi* and blood to the muscles and the flesh. And finally, Spleen *chi* keeps blood in its proper channels.

If the Spleen *chi* itself is deficient, or otherwise not functioning properly, a wide array of physical disorders can result. An overall *chi* deficiency, blood deficiency, or chronic fatigue may occur. The digestion can become poor, and abdominal bloating or diarrhea can follow. The muscles can become weak, and the body thin and emaciated. Heavy menstrual bleeding or other bleeding disorders can occur. Although these varied symptoms have no apparent relationship to one other according to Western medicine, Chinese doctors treat them successfully with acupuncture and herbal treatments to the Spleen, and appropriate dietary and lifestyle changes.

The Spleen *chi* is most easily thrown into disorder by improper diet and eating habits. Poor quality food, heavy or greasy food, meals eaten in a hurry or at the wrong time of day, food allergies, or a diet improper for an individual's constitution can all disrupt the Spleen and cause any of the above symptoms. Once the Spleen *chi* is deficient, a vicious cycle can occur: the deficient Spleen produces less *chi*, overall *chi* deficiency develops, and the Spleen *chi* then has even less *chi* with which to do its work. This is why great emphasis is placed on diet and digestion in Chinese medicine and other systems of natural healing. In my own herbal practice, I have often seen run-down patients regain their strength and health with nothing more than dietary changes and simple Western herbal digestive formulas.

One of Asian ginseng's primary functions is as a tonic to Spleen *chi*, the power supply of the Spleen. Ginseng directly benefits overall *chi*, and also tones up the *chi*-generating properties of the Spleen. But in order for ginseng to do its work, the digestive system must be in shape. In Chinese practice, digestive herbs such as poria, licorice, jujube dates, or ginger are included in a formula with ginseng to ensure this. Other Chinese herbs, such as atractylodes, are even better tonics to Spleen *chi* than Asian ginseng, but these other herbs do not have the wide-ranging effects that ginseng does on overall *chi* and on the other organ systems.

The Lung

Asian ginseng is also a tonic to the Lung. The Lung takes in external *chi* from the air and mixes it with *chi* derived from food by the Spleen. The Lung also circulates protective *chi* to the surface of the body, where it controls sweating and the immune system at the surface of the body. The rhythmic motion of the Lung ensures the rhythmic circulation of *chi* throughout the body. The Lung also has a role in disseminating moisture throughout the body, particularly to the skin. It also drives liquids down toward the Kidney.

Thus, if Lung *chi* — the vital power that allows breathing and the dissemination of protective *chi* and moisture — is deficient, improper circulation can cause deficient or stagnant *chi* in other parts of the body. An individual may develop poor resistance to colds and flu, or may sweat spontaneously with little exertion. The skin may become very dry. A chronic cough or shortness of breath may develop. Even urinary problems may develop.

Part of Asian ginseng's great power as a *chi* tonic comes from the fact that it benefits both the Spleen and the Lung, the two main partners in *chi*-generation. Codonopsis, a ginseng substitute used in China, also acts as a tonic for these two organs, and some practitioners hold that it does so even better than ginseng. Astragalus, a Chinese herb with growing popularity in the U.S. as an immune stimulant, is a premier

Lung tonic that strengthens the circulation of protective *chi* by the Lung. Asian ginseng's effect on the lungs can be readily experienced; shortly after I take ginseng, I feel my breathing become deeper and more relaxed. American ginseng is especially good for this effect.

The Heart

Another benefit of Asian ginseng, which is not shared by the other tonics to the Spleen and Lung, is its beneficial action on the Heart. In the Chinese system, the functions of the Heart include those of the physical heart organ and the arteries; the Heart circulates the blood. But just as important, the Heart pattern includes the conscious mind. "The Heart contains the Spirit," according to classical texts. When the Heart is disturbed, physical symptoms such as palpitations or irregular heartbeat may occur. Mental symptoms such as clouded mind, anxiety, restlessness, insomnia, or excessive dreaming may also appear. In fact, the mental symptoms even without the accompanying physical symptoms will be treated through the Heart in Chinese medicine. Heart symptoms often accompany deficiency syndromes, and ginseng has a specific calming effect on the mental symptoms.

The Liver

The Liver is not directly affected by ginseng, except through its overall *chi*- and blood-building properties. Other tonic herbs I'll describe in Chapter 13 have specific effects on this organ, however, so I'll describe it here. The Liver is described in one Chinese classical text as "the general of the army," because it directs the *chi*, the blood, and even the emotions to flow in an orderly manner. When the Liver is not operating properly, *chi* or blood may become stagnant or erratically excessive, and a person might feel emotionally "stuck" as well. Frustration, anger, and outbursts of rage are common symptoms of a Liver disharmony.

The Liver has a smoothing effect on the flow of *chi*, blood, and emotions. An analogy for this smoothing function is a high-quality surge protector for a computer. Electricity can come from an outlet in an uneven flow, rising and falling as other appliances come on or off, as the power in the electrical grid of the city fluctuates, or when lightning strikes. A surge protector smoothes out these fluctuations to ensure an even flow of current to the sensitive elements of the computer. The human body may not be as vulnerable to destruction as a computer, but a wide variety of symptoms may appear if the Liver's regulating function is not working properly.

The Liver also affects digestion by controlling the flow of bile through the Gall Bladder, and it affects blood flow to the periphery of the body during activity and back to the internal organs during rest.

It is important that the Liver be functioning properly if you want to use ginseng or other tonic herbs. Otherwise, it could be like sending a spike of electricity to a computer with a malfunctioning surge protector. Anger, frustration, and tension are common side effects in people who use ginseng improperly. Herbs to benefit the liver are often included in *chi* and blood tonic formulas to aid their effectiveness.

The Kidney

Understanding the Kidney is central to understanding the action of yin and yang tonic herbs, two categories I'll explain in Chapter 13. These herbs are most often used to treat sexual weakness, lower back pain, and premature aging, among other symptoms. According to modern medical texts, Asian ginseng does not directly affect the Kidney, but its reputation as a sexual tonic, stress-reliever, and metabolism-enhancer indicate that it influences the Kidney indirectly. Ginseng, or one of its substitutes, is often included in formulas to strengthen the kidney function.

The Kidney is considered to be the seat of life. It governs reproduction, as well as the growth, maturation, and maintenance of the entire body and of each organ system. The heat of the Kidney is the source of metabolic fire that rules both water balance and overall metabolism. These functions correspond to the actions of the hypothalamus, adrenal, and pituitary glands in Western medicine. People with deficient Kidney function may become cold or may develop water imbalances or reproductive disorders. The Kidney works with the lungs to control breathing; Kidney deficiency can sometimes cause shortness of breath or chronic cough. The Kidney also rules the development and health of the bones; bone disorders such as osteoporosis are treated through the Kidney in Chinese medicine. Because the Kidney also governs the ears and the hearing, deafness and tinnitus are treated through this organ.

Many of the normal signs of aging, such as weakened hearing, frail bones, greying hair, low metabolism, and feeling cold are due to the natural decline of Kidney function toward the end of life. If these signs appear early, an Oriental doctor will select tonic herbs and acupuncture treatments that affect the Kidney. The Kidney can easily be injured through such activities as overwork, overindulgence in sex, and staying up late at night. Asian ginseng's reputation as an anti-aging and endurance-building herb is based on its indirect action on the Kidney. Steamed ginseng, which has a red color and more heating properties than unprocessed ginseng, is a direct tonic to the Kidney fire. Other tonics, such as *he shou wu* (Fo Ti in the West), affect the Kidney directly and also have reputations as sexual restoratives and longevity promoters.

THE CYCLE OF *CHI* IN THE ORGAN SYSTEMS

In Chapter 3, I discussed lifestyle and recommended that you consume a substantial part of your daily caloric intake early in the day and get good rest at night. Now that we've seen something about the Chinese organ systems and organ *chi*, I can further explain these recommendations.

The *chi* in each of the Chinese organ systems peaks at a certain time each day, and is at its lowest point at the opposite time of day (See Table 5.2). The organs that support digestive function and activity have the peak of their organ *chi* between 7:00 a.m. and 7:00 p.m., while the *chi* of the organs that support rebalancing and regeneration of the system peak in the opposite hours. The best time for digestion and for production and circulation of *chi* is from 7:00 a.m. to 1:00 p.m. Thus, the Chinese have a saying: One should eat like a king for breakfast, a prince for lunch, and a pauper for dinner. The best time to take some hard-to-digest tonic herbs, especially blood tonics, is between 9:00 a.m. and 11:00 a.m., when the spleen *chi* is at its peak. The Spleen function has fallen below average by 4:00 p.m. or 5:00 p.m., so this is a good time to eat like a pauper. On the other hand, sleeping during the

TABLE 5.2
THE CYCLE OF *CHI* IN THE CHINESE ORGAN SYSTEMS

Organ System	Function
5:00 a.m. to 7:00 a.m. Large Intestine	Completion of the night's regenerative function. Preparation for evacuation. Psychological release through dreaming. Good time for meditation or prayer in preparation for the day.
7:00 a.m. to 11:00 a.m. Stomach and Spleen	Best time to eat. Peak time for digestion of food and for its transformation into *chi* and blood. Nutrients are circulated to the muscles and flesh for the day's work.
11:00 a.m. to 3:00 p.m. Heart and Small Intestine	Peak time for circulation of *chi* and blood. The conscious mind is also at its peak. Worst time of day to sleep. The Spleen function is declining. Best time to finish lunch, with lunch and breakfast together making up most of the caloric intake for the day.

day, eating late, and staying up at night, when the organ systems are trying to regenerate the body, depletes the *chi*.

Many people will say that this cycle does not fit their natural rhythm. However, it's entirely possible that their habitual rhythms result from imbalances of the organ systems. Poor appetite during the daytime hours can be due to Spleen deficiency rather than to an innate hunger clock. Likewise, nocturnal habits and insomnia can be due to imbalances in the regenerative organs. The *chi* of the Heart, the organ likely to be deficient in cases of insomnia or mental unrest, is at its low ebb from 11:00 p.m. to 1:00 a.m.

TABLE 5.2 *continued*

Organ System	Function
3:00 p.m. to 7:00 p.m. Bladder and Kidney	The Kidney's metabolic fire is at its peak, and Spleen function has declined. Good time to finish work, take a nap, meditate or pray, and eat a light meal.
7:00 p.m. to 11:00 p.m. Pericardium and Triple Burner	Good time for light activity and mental pursuits. The time for metabolic balancing and regeneration begins. Best time to review the day and go to bed. Spleen function is at its lowest ebb.
11:00 p.m. to 3:00 a.m. Gallbladder and Liver	Best time to be asleep. Activity during this time draws blood away from the Liver and internal organs and inhibits regenerative functions.
3:00 a.m. to 5:00 a.m. Lung	The Lung regenerates the immune function and supports the restorative work of the Liver. Poor time to be awake.

CONCLUSION

Many of the tonic herbs I'll describe in Chapter 13 are specific organ tonics. Their action is mainly on one or two organ systems rather than on the whole system. In that chapter, I'll list which organs each herb affects; you are now prepared to understand what that means in Chinese medicine. We've now seen a large part of the "elephant" of Chinese medicine. In the next chapter, I'll explain specifically how the Chinese use both Asian and American ginseng.

CHAPTER 6

HOW THE CHINESE USE GINSENG

Herbalism in China includes folk herbalism, self-medication with patent medicines (a rough equivalent of over-the-counter medicines in this country), the herbalism of acupuncturists and others using the formal tradition of Chinese medicine, and herbalism as practiced in modern hospitals, often by doctors with dual degrees in conventional and traditional medicine. These areas all may overlap, but I'll use these divisions to show how the various groups use both Asian and American ginseng.

GINSENG AS A HOUSEHOLD MEDICINE

The knowledge of Asian ginseng and how to use it is common in most households in China. Families know, for instance, that ginseng builds *chi*, moistens a dehydrated system, is used for deficiency conditions, is not appropriate for the young, and is contraindicated when a person shows signs of heat or has an acute illness. Ginseng is used specifically for conditions of weakness and low energy—especially by those over 40 years old—and to aid recovery after fever and illness. It might also be used as a general tonic for older people even when they are in good health, especially in the winter months (in the summer it may be too warming). The Chinese may also use ginseng to enhance spiritual pursuits and meditation. It has been known to "increase wisdom" since before the time of the earliest Chinese texts.

Families may have their own stash of ginseng roots, which are expensive in the third-world economy of China. Elders are highly respected in the Chinese culture, and the treasured roots may be reserved for their health crises.

The ginseng roots are typically prepared in water or liquor along with a few jujube dates. I'll explain how to do this yourself in Chapter 15. Another method of preparation is to steam the root, cut it into thin slices, and eat a few slices a day.

Ginseng Gifts

The roots are so highly valued that they are often given as gifts. It is a sign of esteem and respect to give a well-formed root to a superior, a good customer, or an honored guest. I heard the story of an American teacher who spent some time teaching English in a Chinese village as an unpaid service. When it came time for her to leave, the village elder presented her with a beautiful cloth-wrapped wooden box. Inside was a ginseng root. It is possible that this cultural aura placed on the roots inflates their value far above their actual medicinal value.

Patent Medicines

While the roots themselves are expensive, a variety of lower-priced Chinese patent medicines, extracts, and teas containing ginseng are available through shops and are widely consumed in China. You can find many of these products in Chinese and Korean stores in the U.S. In the next section of this book, I will describe several of them and tell you how to order them. These products are much weaker than the whole ginseng roots; the commercial teas probably contain very little ginseng at all. The better extracts are made from the least valuable ginseng roots and vary in quality, but they have a definite mild tonic effect. Some popular extracts use ginseng alone or in combination with other herbs, such as astragalus or royal jelly.

GINSENG IN TRADITIONAL MEDICINE

Traditional Chinese medicine, which uses herbs, acupuncture, diet, lifestyle changes, and exercises as its main tools, exists as a system of medicine parallel to conventional medicine in China. Some hospitals use only traditional methods. Overlap between the two systems exists, because even in modern conventional hospitals some traditional methods are used.

Formal Chinese medicine actually uses very little ginseng, because the herb codonopsis, which I'll describe in detail in Chapter 13, is routinely substituted for ginseng in all classical formulas except those used in emergency situations. This doesn't reflect a devaluing of ginseng, but rather its high cost, as well as the effectiveness of codonopsis. Historically,

TABLE 6.1
THE FOUR GENTLEMEN FORMULA

For overall *chi* and Spleen *chi* deficiency		
Herb	Amount	Action
Ginseng	3–9 grams	*chi* tonic, moistens dryness, tonic to Spleen and Lung, calms the Heart
Atractylodes	6–9 grams	Spleen tonic, Stomach tonic
Poria	6–9 grams	Spleen tonic, dispels abdominal distension
Honey-fried licorice	3–6 grams	*chi* tonic, strengthens digestion, disperses the action of the formula into all 12 meridians

Asian ginseng was used in traditional medicine in formulas. I'll describe the most important formula below.

The Four Gentlemen

The Four Gentlemen formula has appeared in classical Chinese texts since about A.D. 1100. This is a classical formula for tonifying the *chi*.

In modern practice, codonopsis is substituted for ginseng, at two to three times the dosage. Codonopsis acts as a tonic for the Spleen and Lung and also moistens dryness. The formula, like all *chi* tonic formulas, focuses on the Chinese Spleen. I discussed in detail the importance of the Spleen to *chi* in Chapter 5. The transformative function of the Spleen is the source of *chi* and blood in the body. Atractylodes is included because it is even more powerful as a Spleen tonic than ginseng, and because its bitter flavor also tones up the

Stomach. Poria is included because abdominal bloating so often accompanies Spleen deficiency; it reduces such bloating, and is also diuretic. Licorice, when fried in honey, is a warming *chi* tonic and improves digestion. It has a tendency to cause bloating itself, so it goes well with the Poria, which has the opposite tendency. The two balance each other, while aiding the deficient digestion to handle the other herbs in the formula. Licorice is also understood in Chinese medicine to "enter" all the 12 acupuncture meridians. It is included in many formulas to "guide" the effects of the formula throughout the entire body.

Chinese formulas are very versatile; notice that the amounts of the herbs in the formula are given in ranges rather than fixed doses. These are the dose ranges used by modern practitioners. The Chinese herbalist can modify the proportions of the herbs to fit the individual patient. He or she might use more poria and less licorice, for instance, if there is abdominal bloating, more or less ginseng depending on how deficient the patient's *chi* is, and more or less atractylodes depending on the extent of Spleen deficiency.

Chinese formulas are also modified by adding more herbs to them. This Four Gentlemen formula is the root formula for dozens of other *chi* tonic formulas, each adapted to one of the many variations of *chi* or blood deficiency and to the state of the organs in the individual patient. See Table 6.2 for more examples.

Other Formulas

Asian ginseng, or its codonopsis substitute, is included in dozens of other classical formulas used to treat a wide variety of conditions and diseases that result from deficiency.

TABLE 6.2
SOME VARIATIONS OF THE FOUR GENTLEMEN FORMULA

To treat deficiency accompanied by diarrhea and vomiting
in children:

Ginseng	7.5	grams
Atractylodes	15	grams
Poria	15	grams
Honey-fried licorice	3	grams
Aucklandia	6	grams
Agastache	15	grams
Pueraria	15–30	grams

For intermittent fevers with spontaneous sweating and cold signs:

Astragalus	12–24 grams
Ginseng	9–12 grams
Atractylodes	9–12 grams
Honey-fried licorice	3–6 grams
Dong quai	6–12 grams
Citrus peel	6–9 grams
Cimicifuga	3–6 grams
Bupleurum	3–9 grams

For chronic cough from deficiency with heat signs:

Ginseng	60 grams
Poria	60 grams
Honey-fried licorice	150 grams
Gecko lizard	1 pair
Mori alba	60 grams
Almond kernel	150 grams
Fritillaria	60 grams
Anemarrhena	60 grams

Source: Bensky and Barolet

Table 6.3 shows the wide range of possible conditions that can have deficiency as a contributing factor. In most cases, ginseng is not included to treat the disease directly, but to provide the energy in the system for the other herbs to do their work.

More Information About Patent Medicines

I mentioned earlier the patent ginseng preparations that many Chinese people purchase in shops. A wide variety of such medicines exist, and they are used in traditional medical practice as well as by the lay public. Go into any well-stocked Asian store, and you can find dozens of these brightly packaged products. Many are based on classical formulas. They are more complex to take than American over-the-counter medicines, however. You might take an aspirin for a headache or a decongestant for a cold. But the cold medicine you select in an Asian shop might be for either "wind-cold" or "wind-heat," terms the Asians understand. In most such shops, the proprietor or a key employee is an expert herbalist, and will give consultations. Lay self-prescription of herbs thus meets traditional medicine in such stores.

The many patent remedies based on classical formulas that once called for Asian ginseng typically contain codonopsis today. The Chinese patent medicines are usually made from the lowest grades of herbs, with the better quality herbs sold in bulk at higher prices. Many American companies now make the equivalent of these patent medicines, but from higher-grade herbs. Some of these formulas actually contain high-quality Asian ginseng instead of the codonopsis substitute. I'll describe some of these products in Appendix A, and tell you how to obtain them.

TABLE 6.3
SOME HERBAL COMBINATIONS WITH GINSENG
IN TRADITIONAL CHINESE MEDICINE

Ginseng with *Vitex rotundifolia (man jing zi)* berries and astragalus (*huang qi*) for eye disease, tinnitus, deafness, and dizziness from deficiency conditions.

Ginseng with ginger root (*gan jiang*) and pinellia (*ban xia*) for vomiting due to deficiency and cold.

Ginseng with cinnamon (*rou gui*) and rehmannia (*shu di huang*) for heart palpitations due to deficient Heart and Kidney.

Ginseng with prepared aconite (*fu zi*) for the profuse sweating, icy cold extremities, shortness of breath, and other symptoms associated with shock.

Ginseng with atractylodes (*bai chu*) for anorexia, diarrhea, vomiting, abdominal distension, and fatigue from deficient Spleen.

Ginseng with schizandra (*wu wei zi*) and Ophiopogon (*mai men dong*) for shortness of breath and spontaneous sweating associated with deficient *chi* and yin.

Ginseng with rehmannia (*shu di huang*) and asparagus root (*tian men dong*) for fever, thirst, irritability, shortness of breath, and a dry, red tongue from deficient *chi* and yin.

Ginseng with astragalus for general debility, decreased appetite, fatigue, and spontaneous sweating from deficient *chi*.

Ginseng with *huang jing* polygonum for weakness and debility, decreased appetite, fatigue, and emaciation as the aftermath of prolonged illness or as the result of chronic wasting disease.

Ginseng with *he shou wu* polygonum, angelica (*dong quai*), carapax (*bei jia*) and anemarrhena (*shi mu*) for chronic intermittent fever and chills with physical debility.

Ginseng with deer antler (*lu rong*) for palpitations, lower back pain, and decreased or difficult urination associated with severely deficient Heart and Kidney.

TABLE 6.3 *continued*

Ginseng with gecko lizard (*ge jie*), Semen Juglandis regia (*hu tao ren*) and schizandra (*wu wei zi*) for cough and wheezing from deficient Lung and Kidney, and for impotence, decreased sexual function, diarrhea, and frequent urination induced by deficiency.

Ginseng with asparagus root (*tian men dong*) and rehmannia (*shu di huang*) for debility and low-grade fever from deficiency, as in the aftermath of a severe illness.

Ginseng with ophiopogonis (*mai men dong*) and schizandra berries (*wu wei zi*) for profuse sweating, wheezing, increased heart rate, and exhaustion associated with severe deficiency of Heart and Lung, and for excessive loss of fluids in hot weather.

Ginseng with cornus fruit (*shan yu rou*), dragon bone (*long gu*), oyster shell (*mu li*), and aconite (*fu zi*) for profuse sweating from devastated yang with collapsed *chi*.

Source: Bensky and Gamble

Raising the Dead

Asian ginseng is used today in China, as it was in the past, to temporarily revive terminally ill patients. This practice was used with dying Chinese emperors. When it became apparent that the ruler was about to lapse into death, he would receive large doses of ginseng. This would return him to consciousness for a few hours or days so that he could settle state affairs.

As unlikely as such a story might sound to a Westerner, American herbalist and acupuncturist Michael Tierra of Santa Cruz, California, tells of two cases in which he witnessed just such a revival. One man was dying of heart failure, the other of cancer. Each apparently only had days or weeks to live. He prescribed one whole ginseng root a day for each patient. "It brought them out of a comatose state," he says, "noticeable within two or three days." They died as expected, but the ginseng gave them a chance to say final goodbyes to families and to attend to any unfinished business. "No other herb would have done that," says Tierra.

EMERGENCY MEDICINE

Similarly, the Chinese use ginseng in high doses in emergency medicine, for traumatic shock, and for severe chronic diseases. The following formula is a standard in traditional hospitals and emergency rooms in China, sometimes prepared ahead for intravenous use.

Unaccompanied Ginseng Decoction: *du shen tang*

Thirty grams of ginseng (classical formulas called for sixty grams!) decocted with five jujube dates.

This formula is used for life-threatening shock from blood loss. It is used for trauma, wounds, and bleeding after childbirth, and for other severe uterine bleeding. When a person has experienced a trauma, especially if accompanied by blood loss, the body may lose its ability to regulate blood volume. Capillaries (the tiniest of the blood vessels) dilate, and even the normal amount of blood in the body becomes insufficient to fill them. Ginseng is used routinely and effectively in traditional hospitals for such cases.

Ginseng and Aconite Decoction: *shen fu tang*

Ginseng: 12 grams
Prepared aconite: 9 grams

Classical formulas called for 30 grams of ginseng and 15 grams of aconite. The lower amounts above are the doses generally used in hospitals in China. This formula is used for chronic conditionss, such as heart failure or heart attack, that have reached a critical stage, and sometimes for the emergency situations described above. Aconite is an extremely powerful herb, never appropriate for self-medication.

GINSENG AND ATHLETES IN CHINA

Many professional athletes in China use Asian ginseng to improve their performance. During the last Olympics, Chinese women distance runners performed so well that their coach was accused of using drugs to build them up during training. They all passed their drug tests, however, and he said that he had given them nothing more than Chinese tonic herbs. He didn't reveal the formula, but it probably included ginseng. Top Chinese athletes invariably take ginseng and tonic herbs in formulas rather than alone. In Chapter 16, I'll explain in detail how athletes can use ginseng and other tonic herbs.

AMERICAN GINSENG

The Chinese consider American ginseng a different plant with different properties than Asian ginseng; they do not

consider it a substitute for their native variety. Few of the
uses of the two plants overlap. This does not mean that they
do not value it highly. It is a prized medicine in the Chinese
culture. The demand for it in China puts a constant strain
on the American supply and drives the price here to about
$300 a pound—about double the price of Asian ginseng. In
recent decades, the Chinese have begun cultivating their own
American ginseng plants.

According to the eighteenth-century Chinese herbal,
*Ben Cao Gang Mu Shi Yi, Omissions from the Grand Materia Med-
ica* by Zhao Xue-Min, in which it first appeared, American
ginseng tastes like Asian ginseng, but it has cold properties
and is used to generate fluids in dehydrated patients and to
break fevers. This is how it is still used in Chinese medicine
today. It also benefits the lungs and is used to relieve coughs
resulting from Lung *chi* deficiencies. It is also used for loss
of blood, thirst, fever, irritability, and tiredness. Although,
like Asian ginseng, it is considered to be a tonic, none of the
Chinese literature classifies it as a general tonic.

Because of its cooling properties, American ginseng is
popular in the hot climates of southern China and Southeast
Asia, and in the rest of China during hot weather. It will
relieve tiredness, and does not have the contraindication for
heat signs that Asian ginseng does. It will quench thirst due
to hot weather and sun exposure.

Albert Y. Leung, in his book *Chinese Herbal Remedies*,
tells of how he saw the two ginsengs used when he was a
child in China. He was not allowed to take Asian ginseng,
and was told that he was "young and strong and should not
require it [Asian ginseng] to overdo what nature was already
doing" for him. But he remembers taking American ginseng
on many occasions, especially in the summer to cool down.

When one of his sisters had scarlet fever, a condition for which Asian ginseng would be contraindicated because of its heating properties, his grandmother gave her American ginseng to help cool her fever. She recovered with no complications.

CONCLUSION

The stories above about treating terminally ill patients with a whole ginseng root a day to revive them should raise your awareness about the caution necessary when using Asian ginseng, especially in large amounts. If it can so energize a comatose, dying patient, imagine the overstimulation and imbalance that such a dose could cause in a healthy person! In Chapter 7, I'll discuss ginseng abuse, including some cases in which individuals took such large doses.

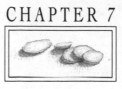

GINSENG
ABUSE

In the late 1970s, the "Ginseng Abuse Syndrome" was big news in herbal circles in the U.S. after an article by that title appeared in the *Journal of the American Medical Association*. A researcher had tracked down 133 long-term users of ginseng, and found that it could cause insomnia and high blood pressure over time. Other symptoms included diarrhea, skin eruptions, and nervousness. The research was so poorly done that it should have been an embarrassment to the editors of the *Journal*. The author did not ask the participants what kind of ginseng they were taking, nor did he identify any of the original herbal material the subjects took. He didn't discuss the fact that the individuals in the study were also taking caffeine, something that was evident from the published data. The adverse effects should have been labeled the "ginseng-caffeine abuse syndrome." In Chapter 11, I will talk more about the problem of taking ginseng and other tonics along with stimulants.

American herbal companies immediately attacked the *Journal* study, circling the wagons around one of their top-selling products. When smoke from the argument clears, however, you can look in any good Chinese medical text, and it will tell you that long-term use of ginseng can lead to insomnia and hypertension, along with heart palpitations, muscle tension, and headache. The *Journal* author, although his science was faulty, had uncovered some basic facts about ginseng.

GINSENG TOXICOLOGY

Overall, ginseng has very low toxicity and is much safer than over-the-counter pharmaceutical drugs you can purchase in any convenience store. Perhaps ten million people in the U.S. consume ginseng regularly, and no truly serious side effects have appeared in the medical literature. In human toxicology studies done in Russia, about 12 ounces of a 3% alcohol solution of ginseng (97% water) caused a mild degree of restlessness. This is a common side effect of ginseng use. Twenty-four ounces produced the symptoms of overdose: systemic rash, itching, dizziness, headache, or fever. In severe cases, bleeding occurred. A single dose, the equivalent of about two quarts of the solution, has caused death.

There are no recorded cases of death from ginseng in this country, despite regular abuse by those who are ignorant of its properties. It is hard to say exactly how the data above translate into doses of either whole roots or of products available in the U.S., because the number of roots in the solutions was not specified in the research. Note that this research showed immediate effects of single doses. Some of these symptoms can appear at lower doses when ginseng is taken for long periods of time.

One or several of the minor symptoms listed above are very common side effects of ginseng overuse. The Chinese know this from several thousand years of observation, and know that they should stop taking ginseng if any of these signs appear. More often, though, they avoid side effects entirely by not taking ginseng when they have excess conditions, heat signs, acute illnesses, or painful conditions. The following lists show contraindications for and possible side effects of ginseng use.

Contraindications for taking Chinese ginseng:

heat signs (see Chapter 4)

signs of excess (see Chapter 4)

high blood pressure (may be okay in mild or moderate cases)

any acute illness, such as colds, flu, or allergy attacks

any painful or inflammatory condition

proneness to nosebleed

excessive menstrual bleeding

pregnancy

youth (ginseng should not be used by children, unless prescribed by a licensed practitioner)

the habitual use of stimulants (caffeine, ephedrine, mahuang)

Possible side effects of regular ginseng use:

diarrhea

headache

heart palpitations

heavy menstrual bleeding

high blood pressure (with prolonged use)

irritability

insomnia
itching
mild fever
muscle tension, especially in the neck and shoulders
nosebleed
rash
red, burning eyes
restlessness

ESTROGENIC EFFECTS

Three anecdotes reporting estrogenic effects in women who took ginseng, including vaginal bleeding in a 72-year-old woman, have appeared in scientific journals. In his book, *The Honest Herbal*, Varro Tyler, Ph.D., says that these reports are inconclusive as to whether ginseng was actually the cause.

A CASE STUDY

A case study of ginseng abuse was submitted to my newsletter, *Medical Herbalism*, by herbalist Jonathan Treasure of Oregon. It involves a man in his forties who had been on a vegan diet (no animal products at all) for about four years. He was run down and depressed, and started taking ginseng to "get going." He took two capsules of eleuthero root (Siberian ginseng) and two vials of Korean ginseng, a liquid form of ginseng available in Asian stores and some health food stores, five days a week. After about three months, he started getting headaches. He kept taking the ginseng, and finally developed a severe nosebleed and an incapacitating headache. Both of these symptoms were observed in the Russian research I described above. He was also drowsy, and had a heavy feeling. These symptoms lasted for four days. He cut his ginseng dose down to three days a week on his own.

This man first saw Treasure about three weeks after the nosebleed. He complained of depression, slow healing of infections, and numbness and tingling in his limbs. The symptoms suggested a vitamin B_{12} deficiency, and other vitamin deficiencies as well. Vitamin B_{12} is not present in a vegan diet. Treasure recommended B_{12} shots, oral B_{12}, and a multivitamin and mineral complex. He also gave the man an herb for the depression, and recommended that he eliminate the ginseng altogether. The patient's symptoms at this point reflected his original underlying condition rather than the ill effects of the ginseng. The patient did not return for his follow-up visit, but Treasure saw him later, and he said that he was "better." He had also started taking the ginseng again!

This patient was definitely deficient, and his problem did not result from taking ginseng when he couldn't use it; such a situation would have led to side effects much faster than the three months they took to show up for him. He is a walking illustration of the point I made in Chapter 3: Don't expect ginseng to take the place of a reasonable diet and lifestyle. His deficiency was due at least in part to his extreme diet, which was not suited to his constitution. He also took the ginseng for too long. A normal course is to take ginseng for six to eight weeks, then take a complete break from it for a week or two. And he took too much; half that dose would have been more appropriate for long-term use. Finally, he did not know the signs of overdose, and kept taking the ginseng after they appeared.

MY STORY

If you take ginseng when you don't need it, adverse effects can show up much faster than they did in the case above. My own story illustrates this perfectly. In the 1980s, before I understood how to use ginseng properly, I was to attend a convention where I would have to sit in board meetings for long hours for several days. The site was at a higher altitude than I was accustomed to. I wasn't particularly deficient, but I thought I'd fortify myself for the stress by taking some ginseng, something I had never done before. I took three or four tablets of a high-quality commercial product each day, along with extra vitamin C. I also drank a lot of coffee while there. I am not the sort who should usually take ginseng, having a robust and active constitution and being prone to develop heat signs easily.

I kept taking the ginseng (and drinking coffee) for a week after the convention. One night, while trying to go to sleep, I noticed that my pulse was racing at about ninety beats per minute and that I had heart palpitations. The men in my family are prone to heart disease, so I went for a complete heart checkup. The doctors couldn't find anything wrong. I finally figured out that the ginseng was causing the symptoms; I stopped taking it, and the symptoms went away. My story illustrates two points: don't take ginseng if you don't need it, and don't take ginseng along with stimulants. I'll discuss the latter point in detail in Chapter 11.

ABUSE ON A GRAND SCALE

I've heard reports of two men who systematically abused ginseng for decades. Their stories show the folly of taking this wonderful medicine in extreme doses. The men were both ginseng traders, with unlimited access to high-quality roots from China. Thus, they were in a position similar to that of drug lords who have unlimited access to cocaine. I heard their stories from one of their colleagues in the ginseng trade. Both men were young when they started taking ginseng, and probably did not need it at all. Both of them took it regularly for 15 to 20 years, sometimes in high doses. One of these men ate a whole $12,000 wild Chinese ginseng root in one sitting!

Both men began to show signs of premature aging while still in their forties. One man's hair suddenly turned completely grey over the course of a single year. The other one, after consuming the whole expensive root, could not function and had to retire from business within a month. He moved to a monastery, where he appeared to age a decade within a year.

In Chinese medicine, the essence of life and growth is contained in the Kidney, and premature aging is seen as a sign of depletion of this essence. It runs down naturally as we age, but excessive exercise and sexual activity can deplete it prematurely. Perhaps these young men used ginseng to support an unnaturally high level of activity and stimulation for decades. They literally "spent" part of their later years prematurely. Their story is not really a warning to the public; most of us couldn't afford to abuse ginseng in that way, and would not be inclined to do so if we could. It's more a call to use ginseng wisely. In an indirect way, it is also a testimonial to the overall safety of ginseng. Despite abuse in a worst-case way, both men remained in apparently normal health for decades before their symptoms appeared.

MISUSE IN AMERICA

For 12 years, in the 1970s and early 1980s, I managed health food stores with herb departments. In that time, I saw many people purchase ginseng. I cannot recall seeing a single buyer who appeared to need it. Most were young, aggressive males who already had plenty of energy, and who wanted to boost their activity level or sexual prowess to unnatural heights. This is the type of person who can most easily develop ginseng abuse syndrome. The Chinese have long believed that ginseng can increase wisdom, but you need a little wisdom in the first place in order to use it properly!

I would especially caution against taking large doses of ginseng. We saw in the last chapter that a 30-gram dose (about an ounce, or one large root) can revive a person from a coma or save them from life-threatening shock. The dose for normal tonic use is a few small slices of such a root. What if the larger dose were taken by a person who is healthy, like the trader in the example above? It could not possibly benefit that person's system, and might disrupt it to a great degree. It would certainly cause major discomfort.

Here are some tips for avoiding the symptoms of ginseng abuse:

- Take ginseng only if you need it.
- Don't take ginseng on an ongoing basis (breaks of a week or two out of every six to eight weeks are appropriate).
- Stop taking ginseng when it has done its work; once you are no longer deficient, or if you begin to show signs of excess, you no longer need it.

• Stop taking ginseng if the side effects listed above begin to appear. The first signs are usually restlessness and tension in the neck and shoulders.

• Don't take ginseng along with caffeine or other stimulants.

• Stop taking ginseng while experiencing transient colds, flu, or other acute illnesses.

SCIENTIFIC RESEARCH ON GINSENG

Asian ginseng is without a doubt the most highly studied medicinal plant in the world. Since the turn of the century, more than 3,000 articles about scientific research on ginseng or its constituents have appeared. Most of the studies have been done in Asia and Russia, and most fall into one of two categories: 1) studies of ginseng's chemical constituents, and 2) studies of the effect of ginseng or its constituents on animals.

Given the high volume of these ginseng studies, there are surprisingly few studies performed on humans, especially double-blind clinical trials—the gold standard of scientific proof. Most of these trials involve Asian ginseng, with very little research available on American ginseng. In this section, I'll review the ginseng research, discuss the constituents of ginseng, and explain how scientists think that ginseng produces the wide variety of medicinal actions attributed to it.

CHAPTER 8

GINSENG RESEARCH

EARLY STUDY OF GINSENG

Scientific research into ginseng began in the mid-nineteenth century, at about the same time that the modern scientific approach was evolving. Because of its fame as a medicine, ginseng attracted the curiosity of some of the earliest medical researchers.

Ginseng's Constituents

The American scientist Garriques isolated a constituent he called "panaquilon" from American ginseng in 1854. The Russian Davydow isolated a similar constituent from Chinese ginseng five years later. By 1915, researchers in Japan and Korea had isolated similar constituents, and identified them as *saponin glycosides*. I'll discuss these substances, which are now called *ginsenosides* or *panaxosides*, later in this chapter. Other substances isolated included a fatty acid and an essential oil.

Early Animal Research

Animal research into ginseng's effects began in the early twentieth century. Stimulating effects on the central nervous system, defensive actions against stress, and metabolism-raising, blood-sugar-lowering, anti-atherosclerotic, and aphrodisiac properties were all demonstrated in animals by the 1920s. Most notably, researchers demonstrated even by this early date that ginseng affects the entire system, not just one organ or mechanism within it. The first published book of ginseng research, the *History of Ginseng*, contained 66 research papers and was published in 1936.

THE RESEARCH OF DR. I. I. BREKHMAN

Ginseng research declined before and during World War II. The real breakthrough in ginseng research came from Russia in the late 1940s and 1950s. Led by the Russian Dr. Itskovity I. Brekhman, a team of scientists performed extensive ginseng experiments on both animals and humans. Their work was an important breakthrough, because they came up with a way to describe the action of ginseng and other tonic herbs in Western terms.

Ginseng's action had been mysterious to most Western scientists, because they had no knowledge of the principles of traditional Chinese medicine. You can't just say that ginseng has "tonic" properties in a scientific article, or that it "builds *chi*." Even if conventional scientists did study Chinese medicine, the results of their work would have to be translated back into Western terms in order to report the results. Perhaps the Brekhman team's most important contribution to ginseng research was to develop a scientific equivalent for the word "tonic."

The Adaptogen Theory

Brekhman and his colleagues coined the term *adaptogen*. An adaptogen is a substance that enables the body as a whole to respond to non-specific stress. A flu shot might strengthen the body's response to the influenza virus, or anti-malarial medicines might protect against malaria, but an adaptogen will protect against a wide range of stressors: sleep deprivation, overwork, physical exercise, trauma, heat, cold, work stress, infection, cancer, and even radiation. An adaptogen does this, not on the strength of its own chemical activity, but by strengthening the body's own innate response mechanisms.

Other properties of an adaptogen, in the Russian model, are that it is non-toxic and that it may be taken as a food. Adaptogenic substances also tend to normalize body functions, enhancing them if they are deficient, and reducing them if they are in excess. Adaptogens are receiving growing recognition among Western scientists as treatments for stress and fatigue.

Publication

In 1957, after conducting a tremendous amount of research on ginseng, including animal and human studies, Brekhman published the results in Russian, in the book *Zen-shen*. He had demonstrated the principle of non-specific resistance by subjecting animals to a wide variety of stresses and comparing the behavior or health of ginseng-treated groups with untreated groups. He also demonstrated improved resistance to stressors and improved athletic performance in humans.

Most of this research unfortunately remains in Russian, and is not accessible to most Western scientists. This has led many Western reviewers to conclude that ginseng is poorly researched.

Brekhman went on to study other Chinese and Russian plants, and discovered adaptogenic properties in the Russian *Eleutherococcus senticosus*, known in the West as eleuthero root or Siberian ginseng. Eleuthero root, although not as versatile or powerful as Asian ginseng, has become a common anti-stress medicine both in Russia and in the U.S.

THE ROLE OF GINSENOSIDES

In the 1950s and 1960s, Japanese and Russian scientists further identified the saponin glycosides that had been discovered earlier in the century. The Japanese Shibata and Tanaka groups found 13 different kinds of saponins in Chinese ginseng, and named them *ginsenosides*. An aromatic compound called "panacene" was also discovered. Most ginseng research since then has focused on studying these isolated constituents rather than whole ginseng root. Many of ginseng's properties were attributed to these compounds.

In the last six years, Korean researchers, using more sophisticated isolation techniques, have discovered that some properties attributed to the ginsenosides were actually due to impurities — other ginseng constituents — in the previous extractions. Korean research today is focusing on these other constituents rather than on the ginsenosides. I will cover ginsenosides and other constituents in more detail in Chapter 9.

SUMMARY OF RESEARCH FINDINGS

Research on the medical uses of ginseng has covered a wide range of health conditions. I will summarize them here in alphabetical order.

Aging

The Chinese have taken ginseng as an anti-aging tonic since before the dawn of recorded medical history. Although it is difficult to design a clinical trial to evaluate an increase in the length of life, research has given some support to the existence of this anti-aging effect. In a variety of studies, scientists have demonstrated that ginseng retards the degeneration of cells, promotes cellular proliferation, and relieves general health problems associated with aging.

Ginseng is also an antioxidant, helping to rid the body of destructive free radicals that scientists believe play an important part in aging. When this evidence is combined with the other effects noted below — enhancing immunity, lowering blood pressure, relieving stress, protecting the liver, counteracting atherosclerosis and diabetes, and generally detoxifying the body — it seems reasonable to conclude that ginseng can extend life.

Alcohol Detoxification

An experiment on alcohol detoxification used healthy male volunteers between 25 and 35 years old as subjects. The men abstained from alcohol and ginseng for a week before the test, then drank 2.5 ounces of 50-proof alcohol for each 140 pounds of body weight (the equivalent of three or four drinks) over a period of 45 minutes. Researchers then measured the levels of alcohol in the men's blood.

A week later, the experiment was repeated, but this time the equivalent of 3 grams of ginseng, in extract form, was added to the alcohol for each 140 pounds of body weight. This time, 70% of the men had blood-alcohol levels in a range 30–50% lower than in the previous test. Animal experiments have revealed similar results, and also demonstrated how ginseng increases alcohol detoxification: it increases the activity of alcohol dehydrogenase and aldehyde dehydrogenase, two liver enzymes responsible for alcohol detoxification.

Anemia

Traditional Chinese practitioners use ginseng to treat anemia. Scientific experiments have verified this blood-building property of ginseng. In one trial, 50 patients who had been unresponsive to anti-anemia medications were treated with ginseng; they showed a rise in their red blood cell count and improvement of the subjective symptoms of anemia. Various studies have also shown that ginseng increases the levels of white blood cells and platelets, blood components responsible for clotting.

Athletic Performance

The first controlled test of the effects of ginseng on humans was conducted in 1948 by Russian scientists. Researcher Dr. I.I. Brekhman gave a ginseng extract to a group of 50 soldiers a few hours before they took part in a three-kilometer run (about two miles). Another 50 soldiers received a placebo: a spoonful of flavored water. The soldiers who took ginseng finished the course in an average of 14 minutes and 33 seconds. The soldiers who got the placebo took, on the average, 53 seconds longer to finish the race. Brekhman commented on the results: "Let us, for a moment, suppose that both groups were carrying batons with important messages . . . those that had drunk ginseng would have delivered their message 45 minutes earlier." Later trials by the Russians showed that some other tonic herbs, including eleuthero root, also positively affected athletic performance.

Subsequent research on humans has demonstrated that ginseng:

- Increases aerobic power and aerobic capacity
- Lowers the peak heart rate on standardized exercise tests
- Hastens the return of the heart rate to normal after exertion
- Lessens the increase in lactic acid levels after exercise (lactic acid is responsible for muscle pain after exercise)
- Improves reaction time

Animals also showed improved performance during vigorous exercise after taking ginseng. Research has shown that they:

- Utilize less stored glycogen
- Take longer to reach exhaustion
- Improve in most measures of performance

Cancer (see also Immunity below)

Ginseng is not a cure for cancer, but clinical studies have shown that it can reduce the symptoms of cancer and improve weakened immune systems in cancer patients.

Ginseng can be used alone or in conjunction with anti-cancer drugs to increase their effectiveness or reduce their side effects.

A group of 100 cancer patients, suffering from gastric, colonic, and pancreatic cancer, were treated for three months with a constituent called prostisol isolated from ginseng. In about 75% of the patients, the injections prevented both the recurrence of cancer and the growth of tumors, and improved red blood cell counts and blood measures of immunity.

In another trial with 150 patients suffering from rectal, breast, and ovarian cancer, taking ginseng orally for 30 to 60 days prevented progression of the disease. White blood cell counts and other measures of immunity improved. Ginseng also normalized the body temperature of one patient in the group who had a fever induced by radiation treatments.

In human patients receiving radiation therapy and chemotherapy, ginseng increased the anti-cancer effects of these therapies.

In animal studies, ginseng increased the resistance of animals to cancer-causing agents, and increased the activity of natural killer cells—white blood cells that are especially important in the fight against tumors.

When tumors were implanted into mice, ginseng extracts dramatically improved the response of the immune system, causing a 33–50% reduction in tumor weight.

The Cardiovascular System

Ginseng may improve many aspects of cardiovascular disease, including blood pressure, blood flow to the heart, blood lipid levels, and atherosclerosis.

Blood Pressure   The effects of ginseng on high blood pressure in animals, such as the effects in the central nervous system (see below), are contradictory. Smaller doses increase blood pressure, while high doses decrease it. Don't take this as advice to take a high dose of ginseng if you have high blood pressure, however; animal trials often do not translate well into human clinical experience, and ginseng is considered by the Chinese to be contraindicated in humans with very high blood pressure. Some scientists hold the opinion that ginseng will raise low blood pressure, and lower mildly or moderately elevated blood pressure. This is consistent with the role of an adaptogen; it will help the system to adapt.

In a case study reported by the Russian researcher I.M. Popov, a 56-year-old male patient with high blood pressure and a blood cholesterol level of more than 325 mg-% (the upper range of normal blood cholesterol is 200 mg-%) had failed to respond to any conventional medications. He took ginseng extract twice a day for two weeks, and then once a day for another two weeks. At the end of this time, his blood pressure had returned to the normal range and his serum cholesterol had fallen to 225 mg-%.

Blood Flow to the Heart   Some animal trials have shown that ginseng dilates the coronary arteries, thus increasing blood flow to the heart.

Atherosclerosis   Atherosclerosis is the hardening of the arteries and the formation of plaque that contributes to high blood pressure, heart attack, stroke, and other such conditions. In clinical experiments, ginseng has lowered total blood cholesterol and triglyceride levels — important measures of the risk of atherosclerosis — and increased levels of the "good" HDL cholesterol. Subjective symptoms of athero-sclerosis, such as insomnia, cold extremities, numbness in the limbs, and heart palpitations, also improved after ginseng administration.

Ginseng extracts have also lowered blood lipid levels and fatty deposits in the organs and veins of experimental animals. Pretreatment with ginseng has prevented both weight gain and atherosclerosis in animals fed an extreme high-fat diet.

The Central Nervous System

In animal research, scientists have found that ginseng has a dual effect on the central nervous system. Different chemical substances that normally occur in the brain can either stimulate or inhibit nerve response. The balance of these substances determines whether the system is activated or sedated. Ginseng appears to increase both the stimulating and the inhibiting processes. It has somewhat more stimulating effects in low doses in animals, and more sedating effects in high doses. These high doses in animal trials may not have relevance to the clinical doses in humans. In lower doses, ginseng has about the same stimulating effect as caffeine in animals. In traditional Chinese use, ginseng will both increase alertness and calm anxiety. Nervousness is one of the first signs of overdose in humans.

Diabetes

Ginseng will not cure diabetes, but it can relieve some of its symptoms and help to lower the required insulin doses. Ginseng may be most beneficial in mild and moderate cases of diabetes. In mild cases, ginseng can reduce the level of sugar in both the urine and the blood. In moderate cases, it does not have this effect to any significant degree, but it lessens symptoms such as fatigue, thirst, and reduced sexual desire. Ginseng is not a substitute for insulin, antidiabetic drugs, or a prudent diet.

The Gastrointestinal Tract

Ginseng apparently has a preventive effect against peptic ulcer disease. Research reports are contradictory, however. Some scientists caution against using ginseng in active ulcerative diseases.

Immunity

A long-term, low dose of ginseng increase animals' resistance to disease. It also heightens the inflammatory response to irritants. High doses in animals have the opposite effect.

Extracts of ginseng root also increase the activity of a group of immune cells that engulf foreign organisms. Mice develop higher levels of antibodies to injected foreign blood cells when the mice are pretreated with ginseng.

Learning

During the 1950s, the Bulgarian scientist Vesselin Petkov conducted research into ginseng's effect on learning and cognitive function. In conditioned learning experiments—in which, for example, the experimenter provides a mild electrical shock to an animal after sounding a bell — animals will learn to associate two different stimuli. Later, if the bell is sounded without the shock, the animal will respond as if a shock were about to arrive.

Petkov demonstrated that both humans and animals will learn associations faster when pre-treated with ginseng. He also showed that they will *unlearn* faster; if the experimenter stops providing the second stimulus, ginseng-treated animals and humans will learn to forget it faster than untreated subjects. Petkov demonstrated that ginseng's adaptogenic effects are not only physical, but extend into the realm of psychology and learning as well.

Liver Disorders

In animals, pretreatment with ginseng protects against liver toxins and hastens regeneration of the liver after experimental damage. In humans, ginseng along with conventional treatments improves recovery time in hepatitis-B patients, and prevents acute hepatitis from progressing to the chronic level. Ginseng may also protect the liver from heavy metal poisoning; it increases the excretion of lead, mercury, and cadmium in the urine.

Menopause

In a clinical trial, ginseng powder was given to 83 menopausal patients for 8 weeks. Menopausal symptoms such as hot flashes, weakness, and tiredness were alleviated in 70 of the women.

Metabolism

Ginseng increases the synthesis of proteins and nucleic acids, important markers of the metabolic rate. Ginseng is able to raise the basal metabolic rate of animals that have had their thyroid glands removed. Large doses over short periods of time increase the thyroid activity of rabbits, but long-term doses decrease the thyroid function in rats. Animal studies such as these are not always relevant to human consumption.

Radiation Exposure

Experiments on both animals and humans have shown that ginseng can minimize the effects of radiation exposure. This could have clinical significance for cancer patients undergoing radiation treatment. One of the main effects of radiation exposure is a drop in the number of both red and white blood cells. A group of cancer patients undergoing radiation therapy received ginseng extracts for 30 days. By the end of that time, abnormally low levels of red and white blood cells had returned to normal.

Many animal trials have shown that ginseng can protect against radiation exposure. Red and white blood cell counts, blood clotting factors, and mast cells in the skin (responsible for hypersensitivity reactions), were all restored to some extent in mice exposed to radiation. Recovery from injury to the bone marrow and to organs responsible for red blood cell formation was hastened when mice were given ginseng extracts.

One Japanese researcher, Dr. M. Yonezawa, states that ginseng appears to be the most useful agent available for protection against radiation damage.

Sexual and Reproductive Function

Ginseng has long been used to treat impotence in Asia. Clinical trials have shown that ginseng can increase both sperm production and sperm motility. Some scientists think that ginseng has an estrogenic effect, but a review of the literature concluded that the evidence of this was poor. In many experiments, ginseng was shown to improve the sexual behavior of animals exposed to stress. Ginseng enhances the maturation of the sex organs in both males and females, prolongs duration of coitus, and increases libido and erection. It appears to increase libido through direct action on the higher brain centers.

Impotence   Russian researchers found that ginseng can effectively treat some cases of impotence. Brekhman gave ginseng to 44 patients with impotence who had not responded to any other medication. Twenty-one of those patients recovered completely, and others improved. Popov gave ginseng to 27 impotent patients. Fifteen recovered completely, and nine improved. Other research showed that ginseng helped to alleviate impotence in diabetic patients.

Hormonal Regulation   Animal studies have shown that ginseng can increase the secretion of luteinizing hormone by the pituitary gland. This hormone, in turn, regulates the secretion of testosterone in the male. It has a more complex action in the female, but is a key hormone in regulation of the menstrual cycle and is the main hormone that triggers ovulation. In humans, such hormonal effects are not seen with low doses of ginseng (1 gram/day), but are evident at doses of 3 or more grams per day.

Stress and Fatigue

Most experiments on ginseng and stress have been conducted on animals. Hundreds of such experiments have been published, and the results have been consistent. With ginseng, animals consistently fare better against such stressors as heat, cold, electrical shock, vibration, low atmospheric pressure, and immobilization. In animals, ginseng prevents the deterioration of the adrenals, spleen, thymus, and thyroid—glands that normally become somewhat smaller under stressful conditions. Hens given ginseng maintain egg production better in cold weather (production normally falls with the stress of cold).

A typical symptom of severe stress is disturbance of the sexual drive and sexual cycle. In a series of animal trials, mice were subjected to experimental stress, and then their sexual behavior was observed. As expected, sexual behavior was disrupted. In a group of mice that received ginseng immediately after the stress, however, sexual behavior was near normal.

In humans, ginseng strengthens the body's ability to adapt to temperature changes, and it has a profound antifatigue effect.

Stephen Fulder, Ph.D., of Great Britain tested ginseng's anti-fatigue effects on a group of night-duty nurses.

When the nurses took ginseng extract, they were more alert and felt less tired than when they did not take it. They also scored better on tests of speed and coordination.

Dr. M.A. Medvedev of Russia performed a similar experiment on a group of radio operators who used Morse code. The group that took ginseng did not transmit code any faster, but they made only about half as many mistakes as those who had not taken ginseng.

CONCLUSION

Most of the human trials involving ginseng do not meet scientific standards; they were either isolated studies unverified by other researchers, or the trial design was not of a quality to deliver definitive scientific proof.

However, *The Lawrence Review of Natural Products*, a conservative scientific publication that reviews herbal and other natural medicines, concludes in its monograph on ginseng: "Numerous animal studies have confirmed . . . [ginseng's] . . . adaptogenic effect, and preliminary clinical evidence also indicates this effect is demonstrable in man. However, . . . the proper dose and duration of use remains poorly defined."

In Chapter 13, we'll turn to Chinese traditions for guidance about dosages and duration of treatment.

CHAPTER 9

CONSTITUENTS OF GINSENG

"The effects of ginseng must not be attributed to one or a few active components; they must be the orchestrated effects of a still not completely understood multi-component system."

Florence Lee, Ph.D.,
former Director,
Laboratory of Pharmacology,
Korean Ginseng Research Institute

Ginseng is unusually rich in active constituents. Many medicinal plants have one or a few such constituents, but ginseng may have 30 or more. Its action is due to these many constituents working together, like the instruments in a symphony.

Virtually all pharmacological and clinical research into ginseng's constituents has focused on ginsenosides (also called panaxosides), which were first discovered in ginseng. A number of clinical investigations were conducted in both animals and humans using isolated ginsenosides, and many of ginseng's properties were attributed to them by scientists. In stores today, it is common to find ginseng products

THE CONSTITUENT GROUPS OF GINSENG

saponin glycosides (ginsenosides, panaxosides)
polyacetylenes
alkaloids
polysaccharides
essential oils
fatty acids
steroids
amino acids
peptides
nucleotides
vitamins
choline
starch
pectins
cellulose

"standardized for ginsenosides." More recent research has demonstrated that some of the properties that scientists attributed to ginsenosides actually belong to other constituents of the plant, but no other specific constituents have been demonstrated to account for ginseng's activity.

GINSENOSIDES

Ginsenosides are of a class of chemicals called *saponin glycosides*. These molecules have a non-sugar backbone with one or more sugar molecules attached. The name "saponin" comes from the English word "soap," because isolated saponins form a soapy foam when shaken in a closed container. Most ginsenosides have two sugar molecules attached to this backbone. Many other adaptogenic herbs also have saponin glycosides as constituents, but they differ somewhat chemically from the ginsenosides.

Nomenclature

Individual ginsenosides are differentiated and named for chemical properties in a common analytical test called *thin layer chromatography*. In this test, a strip of chemically sensitive paper is dipped into a sample. Different constituents in the sample have different solubilities, and they travel different distances up the paper as they are absorbed. In thin layer chromatography, the different constituents appear as separate bands of color up the paper. Ginsenosides are all named "ginsenoside R," with a second letter after the R describing, in alphabetical order, their sequence on the chromatography paper. Thus, ginsenosides are named ginsenoside R_a, ginsenoside R_b, ginsenoside R_c, and so on. In some cases, they are further differentiated as ginsenoside R_{a1}, R_{a2}, R_{b1}, R_{b2}, R_{b3}, and so on.

Ginsenosides in Various Ginseng Species

In all, scientists have isolated 28 ginsenosides from Chinese ginseng, 13 from American ginseng, 14 from tienchi ginseng, and 10 from Japanese ginseng. These four species, which have similar but not identical medicinal properties, have many ginsenosides in common, but each has a unique "fingerprint" of its own mixture of ginsenosides. There can even be a difference in the ginsenoside pattern between plants of the same species grown in different locations. A Korean study found slightly different ginsenosides in two samples of American ginseng, one from the U.S. and the

TABLE 9.1
SOME GINSENOSIDES FOUND IN CHINESE AND AMERICAN GINSENG

Chinese	American
Ginsenoside R_{a1}	
Ginsenoside R_{a2}	
Ginsenoside R_{b1}	R_{b1}
Ginsenoside R_{b2}	R_{b2}
Ginsenoside R_{b3}	R_{b3}
Ginsenoside R_c	R_c
Ginsenoside R_d	R_d
Ginsenoside R_e	R_e
Ginsenoside R_f	R_f
Ginsenoside R_{g1}	R_{g1}
Ginsenoside R_{g2}	R_{g2}
Ginsenoside R_{h1}	
Ginsenoside R_o	R_o

other from Canada. Table 9.1 compares some of the ginsenosides present in Chinese and American ginseng.

Ginsenoside Soup

Ginsenosides were first isolated by Japanese researchers in the 1960s. Nearly 20 years of subsequent research pointed to the ginsenosides as the constituents that give ginseng its stress-reducing, anti-fatigue, and other properties. Each of the ginsenosides is a unique chemical, and many of them have very different effects. One ginsenoside raises blood pressure, for instance, and another lowers it. One sedates the central nervous system, and another stimulates it. The actions of ginseng cannot be attributed to any one of them alone, and the various effects of the different elements of this ginsenoside soup may contribute to ginseng's versatility as a medicine.

Scientific Second Thoughts on Ginsenosides

Florence C. Lee, Ph.D., was the director of the Laboratory of Pharmacology at the Korean Ginseng Research Institute during the 1980s. She had previously been on the faculty of St. Louis University Medical School. In her book *Facts About Ginseng: The Elixir of Life*, published in 1992, Dr. Lee says that new research casts doubt on much of the previous research on ginsenosides. The problem came to light when Korean scientists developed better extraction techniques for ginsenosides. The less-refined ginsenoside extractions used in earlier research appear to have contained impurities—non-ginsenoside ginseng constituents that may actually have been responsible for some of the effects attributed to the ginsenosides. Dr. Lee says that, in the wake of these findings, Korean scientists are now shifting their attention to these other components.

Dr. Subhuti Dharmananda, president of the Institute for Traditional Medicine in Portland, Oregon, also mentions this research in his paper "The Ginseng Story," which accompanies an Institute video on ginseng. In one Korean experiment, a team of scientists examined the anti-fatigue action of ginseng, duplicating research done decades earlier by Russian scientists. This test consisted of recording how long it took a group of mice to swim to exhaustion. One group of mice received ginseng in their diet for a period of time before the test. The Koreans matched the results of the earlier Russian trial: mice fed ginseng swam about a third longer than mice on a regular diet. Using highly purified ginsenosides instead of whole ginseng extracts, however, the effect was lost. The Korean researchers mentioned maltol, vanillic acid, salicylic acid, and various phenolic compounds as "impurities" that may have properties previously attributed to ginsenosides. Dr. Lee says that current research in Korea is focusing on polyacetylenic compounds, phenolic compounds, and alkaloids, all of which are present in minute quantities in ginseng.

Traditional Second Thoughts on Ginsenosides

Chinese scientists and clinicians have never accepted the theory that ginsenosides are the only active constituents of ginseng. For instance, although fully aware of ginsenoside research, they do not consider ginsenoside content to be a predictor of medicinal potency.

Zhang Shuchen, Ph.D., is China's foremost ginseng expert, with 30 years of ginseng research experience at Chinese institutions. He is the former head of China's Institute of Traditional Chinese Medicine and Materia Medica. Zhang acts as a consultant to the Jade Research Group, an American consulting firm that develops high-quality Chinese herbal products and employs internationally recognized experts in plant research and formulation. Bill Brevoort, coordinator of the Jade Research Group, says that Zhang does not consider ginsenoside content at all when selecting ginseng roots for quality. Instead, he uses traditional Chinese criteria:

• Density. A lighter root has more potency than a heavier root of the same size. Poorer-quality cultivated roots are much more dense than wild roots.

• Ring pattern. Experts judge the quality of a root based on the pattern of rings on the root bark that encircle it. Rings that are smaller and closer together indicate a better root.

• Man-shape. Some ginseng roots resemble the human figure, appearing to have arms and legs. This is the source of the Chinese name for ginseng—*ren shen*—which means "man-root." The Chinese hold that these well-formed roots have more potency than others.

Says Brevoort, "This may sound like superstition, but after you've eaten 25 to 30 roots selected on those principles, you'll believe it." Brevoort adds that Chinese scientist-consultants working for the National Institutes of Health use these same criteria to select ginseng for scientific studies in the U.S. Chinese researchers, although thoroughly familiar with ginsenoside research, have found no correlation between ginsenoside levels and their traditional methods.

For centuries, the Chinese have attributed ginseng's *chi*-building properties to the central root of the plant, but ginsenoside content is highest in the small rootlets and root hairs that branch off of the main root. It is also high in the leaves. It would seem that if ginsenosides were solely responsible for ginseng's remarkable tonic qualities, the Chinese would value these peripheral parts more. To the contrary, the rootlets—called *shen xu*, literally "root whiskers"—are relatively inexpensive in China. They are trimmed from ginseng roots, then cured in rock candy and used as minor tonics for fever. Likewise, the leaf—called *ren shen ye*, or "ginseng leaf"—is used in China as a minor tonic in the same manner as the root whiskers. According to Albert Y. Leung, Ph.D., in his book, *Chinese Herbal Remedies*, the leaf is considered to have medicinal qualities similar to those of American ginseng, used for reducing heat induced by fever or summer heat.

The fact that these peripheral parts of the plant have medicinal value similar to that of American ginseng indicates that the ginsenosides do play a part in the effects of ginseng. But to say that ginsenosides are the only important active constituents of ginseng is like defining an elephant as an animal with a long trunk. The trunk is important, and the animal wouldn't be an elephant without one, but there's a lot more to the elephant than its trunk. And you need the whole elephant to perform circus tricks.

OTHER CONSTITUENTS

Among the ginseng constituents that apparently were extracted along with ginsenosides in early research were phenolic compounds. This is a large class of chemical compounds that includes the active ingredients in aspirin-like plants, flavonoids such as the bioflavonoids available in health food stores, and blood-thinning coumarin medications. Dr. Lee says that current research in Korea is focusing on these constituents, on polyacetylenic compounds, and on alkaloids, all of which are present in minute quantities in ginseng.

Some other constituents in ginseng are called polysaccharides. These are huge, sugar-like molecules. Plant research around the world has shown that many polysaccharide compounds are potent immune-system stimulants; they are found in such well-known immune-system stimulants as echinacea. They are also found in Japanese immune-stimulating mushrooms, such as ganoderma and shiitake. The polysaccharides also moderate the immune-response that is responsible for auto-immune diseases such as lupus.

CHAPTER 10

How Ginseng Works

Researchers have identified actions of different ginseng constituents throughout the body on many organs and glands. But they cannot explain exactly how these effects occur at a biochemical level. Ginseng's constituents are so diverse that precise knowledge of how it works is beyond the scope of current science. It may even seem impossible that ginseng, a single herb, could have so many physiological effects. But an explanation may lie in the role of hormones in regulating the body, and in ginseng's effects on these hormones.

PRIMARY HUMAN GLANDS

The Hypothalamus

All the aspects of the body that ginseng seems to affect—stress, fatigue, blood sugar levels, blood pressure, body temperature, sexual function, detoxification, and immunity—are regulated by hormones produced in the

113

hypothalamus, the pituitary gland, and the adrenal glands. Among these, the hypothalamus, located in the lower brain, is the controller. The hypothalamus constantly monitors the state of the body as well as external threats to it. It receives input from both the body and the brain. The hypothalamus can monitor hormone levels, blood pressure, water balance, blood sugar, and many other physiological parameters. It will also respond when the subconscious mind perceives a stressful situation. The hypothalamus responds to both mental and physiological stimuli.

The Pituitary and Adrenal Glands

The hypothalamus controls the pituitary gland, which acts like its executive officer and in turn controls functions such as metabolism, appetite, body temperature, and water balance. The hypothalamus coordinates these key functions in a harmonious way, while the pituitary carries out its instructions. The hypothalamus also has a direct controlling influence, without its pituitary intermediary, on sexuality, growth, and reproduction.

One of the most important secretions of the pituitary is a hormone that activates the adrenal glands, the glands responsible for the "fight or flight" reaction. When the brain perceives a threat to survival, the hypothalamus activates the pituitary, which in turn activates the adrenal glands to flood the body with stress hormones. These stress hormones, in turn, instruct the pituitary that they are doing their job, and prevent further stimulation by the pituitary. Scientists call the interaction of these three glands the *hypothalamus-pituitary-adrenal axis*. Although the precise mechanism is not known, some ginseng researchers now assume that the activity of ginseng and related adaptogens is primarily on this hormonal system. The hormones have wide-ranging control-ling effects on the body, and if ginseng can modify them, that would explain its similarly wide-ranging effects.

Ginseng and the Adrenal Glands

Ginseng's relation to the adrenal glands is well documented. Ginseng normally increases resistance to stress, but it loses much of this property in animals if their adrenal glands have been removed. Thus, ginseng may act through the intermedi-ary of the adrenal glands, either directly or through the hypo-thalamus' controlling function. In normal animals under stress, ginseng stimulates production of stress hormones. When the stress stops, however, the adrenals stop produc-ing the hormones faster than in animals who have not taken ginseng. But if stress is prolonged, the adrenals of ginseng-treated animals will conserve the stress hormones in order to prolong endurance. Thus, the overall effect of ginseng and other adaptogens on the adrenals is to make them more effi-cient and more adaptable to stress. Whether these effects are solely on the adrenal glands, or whether the hypothalamus and pituitary are somehow also involved, has not been deter-mined by scientists.

Sensitizing the Hypothalamus

Stephen Fulder, Ph.D., a ginseng researcher from Great Britain, performed an experiment that hints at a possible role of ginseng in sensitizing the hypothalamus to make it more efficient. If this is the case, this single action could explain ginseng's effect on the sex glands (which are directly controlled by the hypothalamus), on the pituitary and adrenal glands, and indirectly on all the target organ tissues that these glands regulate.

In Fulder's experiment, laboratory rats had their adrenal glands and ovaries removed to eliminate any possibility of internal production of stress steroids. They were then divided into two groups, one group receiving ginseng for eight days, and the other receiving a placebo. The animals were then injected with corticosterone, the main stress hormone. The hormone was "tagged" chemically so that the researchers could find out exactly where it went in the body. Among the ginseng-treated rats, up to seven times as much corticosterone was deposited in the area of the brain around the hypothalamus, as compared to the placebo group. The hypothalamus normally has a feedback loop for corticosterone; when it detects elevated levels, it takes action to balance them. Ginseng may sensitize the hypothalamus to this feedback loop, increasing the efficiency of its stress-controlling function. Fulder hypothesizes that this "priming" of the hypothalamus initiates hormonal secretions which also improve the efficiency of the brain.

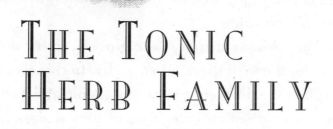

THE TONIC
HERB FAMILY

The oldest book of Chinese medicine lists 365 herbs, and classifies them according to three grades. The lowest grade of herbs dispels disease. The middle grade corrects imbalances in the body. The highest grade—the one to which ginseng belongs—nourishes life itself. These are the tonic herbs, many of them classified as adaptogens in Western scientific terms. If you are thinking of taking ginseng, you would do well to learn about these other herbs. Some other members of the tonic family may be better suited to your particular kind of deficiency than ginseng. One of them, codonopsis, is often used as a ginseng substitute, and costs only about one-tenth as much. Another, dong quai, is a warming blood tonic and a renowned women's herb; in China, it is probably consumed more than any other tonic herb. Learning about these other herbs will also help you to identify them in tonic formulas widely available in health food stores.

The Chinese usually take ginseng in formulas with at least one of these other herbs. In this section, I'll explain the difference between a tonic and a stimulant, outline the four categories of tonics, show you the principles behind tonic formulas, describe the most important members of ginseng's tonic family, and suggest some simple combinations or formulas you might take, either with or without ginseng.

CHAPTER 11

TONICS VS. STIMULANTS

Tonics and stimulants may seem closely related, because they both provide a boost of energy. However, the habitual use of stimulants, including caffeine, guarana (another name for caffeine), ma huang, and ephedrine, is incompatible with the use of ginseng or other tonic herbs. Although stimulants and tonics may both seem like "uppers," their effects are actually opposite to each other. The long-term effect of a stimulant is to exhaust and depress, which can more than cancel out the beneficial effects of a tonic.

The distinction between stimulants and tonics is important; many people with *chi* deficiency who medicate themselves with caffeine or other stimulants end up with less *chi* than they started out with. Taking a tonic is like putting money (*chi*) in the bank. Taking a stimulant is like withdrawing the money; at some point, your account becomes overdrawn. If you continue to spend *chi* without replenishing it, the consequence can be "energy bankruptcy"—severely depleted *chi*. A *chi*-building program, including tonic herbs and other lifestyle changes, is like starting a savings plan; if you're in debt and overdrawn, it's best to cut up your credit cards (stimulants) and start a more rational plan for saving.

Tonics and stimulants do not simply cancel each other out. Taken together, they can create great disharmony and tension in the body. Stimulants such as those mentioned above provide a short-term boost of energy which, when added to the effect of a *chi*-tonic herb, can create strong temporary overstimulation in one organ system or another. A typical result could be tension, heightened insomnia, or high blood pressure. In Chapter 7, I mentioned a Western scientist who identified a number of adverse effects in individuals who took ginseng and caffeine together habitually.

CAFFEINISM

To demonstrate this *chi*-depleting effect of stimulants, I'll use the example of caffeine. "Caffeinism"—the overuse of coffee and tea—was recognized as a medical condition in turn-of-the-century American medical books. Over the last hundred years, our society has turned to caffeine consumption as a normal activity, and lost sight of the consequences of habitual use. On average, Americans consume the caffeine equivalent of one to three cups of coffee a day, coming from coffee itself, soft drinks, or pep pills. Since many people do not take any caffeine at all, this means that many people take much more than this average. About ten percent of the population consumes the equivalent of 18 or more cups of coffee a day. Many people who would be diagnosed with deficient *chi* by a Chinese practitioner, or with stress-related chronic anxiety by a medical doctor, are actually suffering from caffeinism.

The list below shows the symptoms of chronic caffein-ism. Refer to Chapter 2, and notice that these are identical with the symptoms of deficient *chi* and blood. Note that coffee in particular, which contains irritating organic acids, also impairs the digestive system. Gastrointestinal symptoms of chronic coffee consumption include acidity, dyspepsia, bitter and sour belching, flatulence, and constipation. The digestive system is the main source of *chi* in the body, and this irritation further inhibits the production of *chi*. If you have these symptoms and you consume caffeine regularly, try cutting it out completely and see if the problems go away. Table 11.2 shows the quantities of caffeine in various products.

Symptoms of Caffeinism

Symptoms resembling deficient *chi*:

physical exhaustion
muscular weakness
mental exhaustion
dejected spirits
dull, expressionless features
poor digestion
difficult breathing

Symptoms resembling deficient blood:

pale skin
dizziness
insomnia
nervous palpitations
emaciation
mental fatigue

TABLE 11.1
CAFFEINISM AND CHRONIC ANXIETY

Some Symptoms of Caffeinism*	Some Symptoms of Chronic Anxiety**
anxiety	apprehension
tremors	trembling
insomnia	insomnia
nervous irritability	nervousness
hysteria	irrational thinking
heart palpitations	heart palpitations
mental confusion	difficult concentration
muscular weakness	motor weakness
physical exhaustion	chronic fatigue
headaches	headaches

*King's American Dispensatory, 1898
**Merck Manual, 1992 edition

Caffeinism and Anxiety

Table 11.1 compares the symptoms of caffeinism with the conventional diagnosis of chronic anxiety, one form of "stress" in lay terms. Conventional medical texts do not even suggest asking patients with these symptoms if they drink coffee, drink caffeinated drinks, or take caffeine pills. Instead, the doctor will usually prescribe a sedative like Valium, adding potentially addictive drug intoxication to the existing problem of caffeinism.

You don't need to take a lot of caffeine in order to get the symptoms listed in Table 11.1. Some of us might get away with a few cups of coffee or its equivalent per day, but individuals can develop symptoms of caffeinism even from this amount. In one scientific study, patients with anxiety disorder rated their symptoms on a standard test. Their levels of anxiety and depression correlated directly with the amount of caffeine they consumed. Another group of 6 anxiety patients, who consumed the caffeine equivalent of 1.5 to 3.5 cups of coffee per day, cut their intake to zero; within 12 to 18 months, 5 of the 6 were symptom-free.

About 200–300 mg of caffeine a day is the threshold for addiction. Regular use of more than this will result in withdrawal symptoms: headache, weakness, and mental confusion. Symptoms of *chi* deficiency and anxiety can be brought on by 150 mg of caffeine a day.

MY STORY

I stopped drinking coffee four years ago. Prior to that, I had a five-cup-a-day habit and considered it an occupational hazard of being a writer. It was an instant cure for writer's block: one cup of coffee and the words would flow. I found that I would become mentally exhausted after about 45 minutes of writing, and would have to either drink a cup of coffee or

TABLE 11.2
CAFFEINE CONTENT OF FOODS AND DRUGS

8-ounce cup of coffee:	80–130 mg caffeine
strong coffees available in many coffee shops:	200 mg
8-ounce cup of caffeinated tea:	50–70 mg
12-ounce caffeinated soft drinks:	35–60 mg
4 ounces of chocolate:	60 mg
pep pills:	100–200 mg per tablet
pain relievers:	32–65 mg per tablet

take a long break. Eventually, the coffee gave me chronic digestive pain, and I was so run down and nervous that I had to stop.

For a few days after stopping, my energy level was so low that I couldn't do anything at all. I remained "wiped out" for about three weeks. Soon I noticed that, without the coffee, I could write for two hours without a break. The coffee had been creating the problem that I was using it to solve! I noticed during the three-week withdrawal that I had to either take a late-afternoon nap or start drinking coffee again; I couldn't stay awake. I still take that nap now, four years later. I had been using coffee, a *chi*-depleter, as a substitute for what remains for me a natural time of rest and *chi*-cultivation.

MA HUANG, EPHEDRA, EPHEDRINE

Ma huang is another famous Chinese herb, but it is a stimulant rather than a tonic. It is much more potent than caffeine. *Ma huang (Ephedra sinensis)* is the original source of ephedrine, a common ingredient in allergy medicines, weight-loss products, and pep pills. It has a legitimate medical use in the treatment of asthma and allergies, but its use as a stimulant or weight-loss product is unwarranted and dangerous; several deaths have been attributed to its improper use in recent years. It is contraindicated for people with high blood pressure, which is common in overweight people.

I was once teaching a class in Chinese pulse diagnosis at the Rocky Mountain Center for Botanical Studies in Boulder, Colorado. We were measuring the speed of the pulse. Rather than count beats per minute, Western style, Chinese practitioners count the average number of beats per breath.

I have taught this class many times; I have the students take each other's pulses, and then we list the averages on the board. The majority of students always fall around four or five beats per breath, with a few at six beats (a sign of heat in traditional Chinese medicine).

On this particular day, we had the expected cluster around four and five, but we had sixes, sevens, and another cluster between eight and eleven. I was stumped. Then we discovered that someone had brewed a pot of after-lunch tea from a commercial product that contained *ma huang* along with some other herbs. The students with the fast pulses had all consumed the tea, and it had put them into a state resembling that induced by aerobic exercise! This sort of state is completely incompatible with taking ginseng and the other tonic herbs. We repeated the exercise the next day, without the tea, and got the expected pulse frequency.

Habitual use of *ma huang* is extremely *chi*-depleting. I once had a case study of *ma huang* abuse submitted to my *Medical Herbalism* newsletter. A man noticed that he got an energy boost from an allergy medicine. He figured out that the *ma huang* was the key ingredient in the formula, and bought some from an herb store. He brewed a cup or two of it a day, like coffee. After about a month of this, he became so exhausted that one day he could not get out of bed and had to be taken by ambulance to a hospital for an emergency checkup. This case, although extreme, demonstrates the depleting nature of this common stimulant.

TONICS

Tonic herbs, unlike stimulants, do not have instant effects. Think of them as special foods that nourish, rather than as drugs that stimulate. It often takes two weeks or more to see their energy-building effects, and the typical duration of tonic herbal therapy is one to two months. They also do not produce the subsequent "crash" that stimulants do. Taken appropriately and in moderate doses, they will not produce anxiety, tension, or insomnia. In fact, many of the tonic herbs sedate even as they build the energy. The general effect of ginseng, in low doses, is to increase alertness while relaxing emotional tension.

CHAPTER 12

TYPES OF TONICS

I described the symptoms of *chi* deficiency and blood deficiency in Chapter 2, and I provided a checklist for signs of deficiency vs. excess in Chapter 4. In this chapter, I'll describe states of deficiency in more detail.

FOUR DEFICIENCIES AND FOUR TONICS

Chinese medicine recognizes four types of deficiencies for purposes of prescribing tonic herbs: *chi*, blood, yang, and yin. The tonic herbs are classified according to which of these deficiencies they will strengthen. The four deficiencies are not really separate, but they are useful for diagnosis, and they form the basis for preparing tonic formulas. I already described *chi* and blood deficiencies in Chapter 2. Remember that *chi* and blood are closely related; *chi* from the Spleen and Lung build the blood, but sufficient blood is necessary for *chi* to do its work. Signs of these two deficiencies often coexist. *Chi* and blood deficiencies are treated with *chi* and blood tonics, respectively. Because of the interrelation between the two syndromes, either one might be treated with both *chi* and blood tonics.

Yang Deficiency, Yang Tonics

Deficient *chi* can become more severe and progress to a condition called deficient yang. Its main manifestation, in addition to symptoms of deficient *chi*, is signs of cold. Refer to Table 4.2 to review cold signs. Yang deficiency usually involves the Kidney organ, which is viewed in Chinese medicine as the source of heat in the body. In some diagrams of the Chinese organ system, the Kidney is portrayed as a hot cauldron in the lower part of the body. With deficient yang, sexual weakness, lower back pain, weakness in the knees, hearing problems, and brittle bones may become prominent along with signs of cold. Some of these Kidney symptoms overlap with deficient yin, which I'll describe below.

Deficient yang is treated with yang tonics. These herbs (and sometimes animal substances) are warming in nature, and are very potent medicines. They are contraindicated when heat signs are present.

Yin Deficiency, Yin Tonics

Deficient blood involves a deficiency in the volume or quality of the blood. A more serious related condition is "deficient yin," which is a deficiency of body fluids in general. Symptoms of deficient blood are present, but also general dehydration and heat signs. Refer to Table 4.2 to review the signs of heat. The fluids moisten and cool the body, and when they are deficient, the heat becomes prominent with such signs as thirst, dry mouth and lungs, red face, hot hands and feet, insomnia, night sweats, and a rapid pulse. This is a common syndrome in the aftermath of a fever or exhaustion through overwork or prolonged stress.

Yin deficiency is treated with yin tonics. These cooling and moistening herbs restore the fluids and reduce heat. They are contraindicated when signs of cold are prominent.

Complex Deficiencies

Because of the close connection between *chi* and blood, several of these deficiencies may overlap. "Deficient *chi* and blood" is a common Chinese diagnosis, as is "deficient yin and yang." In each case, a combination of the diagnostic signs is present. Complex deficiency syndromes are treated with complex formulas, combining tonics in the appropriate amount for each of the deficiencies to match the intensity of the symptoms. Deficient yang is always accompanied by deficient *chi*, and deficient yin is invariably accompanied by deficient blood. For this reason, *chi* and yang tonics are usually combined in formulas, as are blood and yin tonics. An exception might be when a particular herb tonifies both *chi* and yang, or blood and yin, at the same time.

Ginseng and the Four Deficiencies

Ginseng is known as the king of the tonic herbs, because it can benefit all four of the deficiencies, although skill in avoiding its contraindications is necessary. Ginseng is primarily a *chi* tonic, but it also benefits the blood. It is sometimes used alone or in formulas to treat anemia. Ginseng also "benefits the fluids," alleviating thirst and easing

TABLE 12.1
THE FOUR DEFICIENCIES

Deficiency	Signs in Common	Distinguishing Signs	Tonic Treatment
Chi	pale complexion fatigue low spirits spontaneous sweating low voice weak digestion enlarged tongue	shortness of breath pronounced fatigue loose stool dribbling of urine weak pulse	*Chi* tonics
Yang		aversion to cold cold hands and feet plentiful urine clear urine loose stool with undigested food dark colored tongue slow pulse	Warming yang tonics

dehydration. It can relieve the thirst that accompanies diabetes, for instance. Nevertheless, it is warming, and must be
used with care when dehydration and heat signs are present,
especially for long periods. Steamed red ginseng has very
strong warming properties, and is used as a tonic to both *chi*
and yang. American ginseng, with its cooling properties, is a
premier yin tonic, and moistens dry lungs and throat.

TABLE 12.1 *continued*

Deficiency	Signs in Common	Distinguishing Signs	Tonic Treatment
Blood	emaciation dizziness spots before the eyes heart palpitations insomnia little tongue coat thin, thready pulse	pale complexion pale lips and tongue numbness in the limbs	Blood tonics
Yin		flushed face hot hands and feet dry mouth and throat night sweats premature ejaculation dry, red tongue fast pulse	Cooling and moistening yin tonics

ORGAN DEFICIENCIES

The four deficiencies will present overall signs in the body, but symptoms may appear primarily in one or more organ systems. The tonic herbs each have affinities for specific organs, and are selected in formulas according to the symptoms of the patient. The accompanying box shows some

---

SIGNS OF DEFICIENCY IN THE FIVE MAIN ORGAN SYSTEMS

Spleen   poor appetite
           loose stools
           bloody stool
           abdominal pain relieved with pressure
           weak limbs
           undigested food in stool
           prolapsed organs
           edema
           urinary incontinence

Lung   weak respiration
           frequent colds and flu
           weak cough
           daytime or night sweats
           dry cough
           dry mouth

Heart   palpitations
           insomnia
           irregular pulse, weak pulse
           shortness of breath

---

symptoms of deficiency that can appear in each of the five
major organ systems. These deficiencies might be classified as
yin or yang deficiencies of the organs, depending on whether
overall signs of deficient yin or yang are present. In Chapter
13, I'll describe which organs each of the tonic herbs affects.

TONIC FORMULAS

A basic principal of tonic formulation is that the entire system
of blood and *chi* is tonified. A formula may be weighted heavily in the direction of *chi* and yang, or blood and yin, but

---

Signs of Deficiency in the Five Main Organ Systems
continued

Liver	pain in the side
	dry eyes
	menstrual irregularities
	depression
	nervous tension
Kidney	frequent urination
	dribbling of urine
	low back pain
	weak knees
	premature ejaculation
	low sperm count
	impotence
	sterility
	hearing loss
	tinnitus
	forgetfulness
	frail bones

---

it will contain something to supplement each. This can be accomplished either by selecting herbs with overlapping effects or by including tonics of each type. Table 12.2 shows the overlapping effects of some single tonic herbs. This principle is evident in some of the most common pairings of herbs with ginseng in Chinese formulas:

- Ginseng (*chi* and yin tonic) with astragalus (*chi* and blood tonic);
- Ginseng (*chi* and yin tonic) with *he shou wu* (blood and yin tonic);

TABLE 12.2
THE OVERLAPPING EFFECTS OF SOME TONIC HERBS

Herb	Primary Action	Secondary action
ginseng	*chi* tonic	yin tonic
red ginseng	*chi* tonic	yang tonic (effects about equal)
American ginseng	yin tonic	*chi* tonic (mild)
deer antler	yang tonic	*chi* and blood tonic
astragalus	*chi* tonic	blood tonic
cordyceps	yang tonic	yin tonic (effects about equal)
dong quai	blood tonic	yin tonic (effects about equal)
jujube dates	*chi* tonic	yin tonic
peony	blood tonic	yin tonic (effects about equal)
rehmannia	blood tonic	yin tonic (effects about equal)

- Ginseng (*chi* and blood tonic) with *dong quai* (blood and yin tonic).

Many formulas specifically for blood or yin do not contain *chi* tonics. In this case, because of their overall cooling and moistening nature, other warming herbs are included to ensure good circulation.

The three formulas below, which are readily available commercially in pill form, demonstrate the principles of formulation. All three contain a mixture of *chi* and blood tonics. All three benefit both functions. But the overall effect of the formulas differs due to the type of tonic herbs emphasized in each. The first is more tonifying to the *chi*, the second is balanced, and the third is more tonifying to the blood. Notice that these formulas contain several herbs which are not tonics. These adjuvant, or supplementary, herbs are included to promote digestion or circulation. I'll describe a few of them in detail at the end of the next chapter.

Ginseng Tonic Pills

Ren Shen Yang Rong Wan
A *chi* tonic

ginseng	4 parts	overall *chi* and Spleen *chi* tonic
atractylodes	4 parts	Spleen tonic
astragalus	4 parts	tonic for protective *chi*
citrus peel	4 parts	Spleen tonic; moving adjuvant
rehmannia	3 parts	blood and yin tonic
schizandra	3 parts	*chi* tonic
poria	3 parts	Spleen tonic
jujube dates	6 parts	Spleen tonic
peony	4 parts	yin and blood tonic
polygala	1 part	sedative herb
cinnamon bark	1 part	warming adjuvant
ginger	2 part	warming adjuvant

The above formula actually contains ginseng instead of the usually substituted codonopsis. It is available in Chinese stores as *Ren Shen Yang Yin Wan*. It is also available from McZand Herbals in liquid form as Ginseng Nutritive Formula.

Ten Flavor Tea

Shi Chuan Da Bu Wan
A general tonic for both blood and *chi*

codonopsis	2 parts	*chi* and Spleen tonic
astragalus	2 parts	tonic for protective *chi*
peony	3 parts	yin and blood tonic
atractylodes	3 parts	Spleen tonic

poria	3 parts	Spleen tonic, tranquilizing
rehmannia	3 parts	yin and blood tonic
dong quai	3 parts	yin and blood tonic; promotes circulation
cinnamon	1 part	warming adjuvant
ligusticum	1 part	promotes circulation
licorice	1 part	Spleen tonic; harmonizes other herbs

This balanced formula is a common general tonic in China, where it can be purchased in pill form. It is taken for long periods of time, with a break for a week or two every three months. The pills, which are inexpensive, are available in Chinese stores as *Shih Chuan Ta Pu Wan*, or through the mail from East Earth Tradewinds as *Shih Chuan Da Bu Wan*. The McZand company produces this formula in liquid form, in a product called Ginseng and Tang Kuei Ten Formula.

Women's Precious Pills

Fu Ke Ba Zhen Wan
A blood and yin tonic formula

dong quai	6 parts	yin and blood tonic
rehmannia	6 parts	yin and blood tonic; promotes circulation
codonopsis	4 parts	*chi* and Spleen tonic
poria	4 parts	Spleen tonic
atractylodes	4 parts	Spleen tonic
peony	4 parts	yin and blood tonic
ligusticum	3 parts	promotes circulation
licorice	2 parts	Spleen tonic; harmonizes other herbs

This formula, although containing some *chi* tonics, has more weight on the blood and yin tonic side. It is available in Chinese stores or from East Earth Tradewinds or the Institute for Traditional Medicine as Women's Precious Pills. K'an Herbals sells an excellent variation of this formula as Women's Precious; it contains high-grade herbs, including ginseng (instead of codonopsis) and several other herbs.

CONCLUSION

In the next chapter, I will describe 32 tonic herbs. For each one, I will suggest some simple combinations that you might use, following the principles above.

CHAPTER 13

THE TONIC HERBS

In this chapter, I'll say more about Chinese and American ginseng, and then describe 32 more tonic herbs. Some of these herbs may be taken by themselves. More often they are used in formulas, often including ginseng or its most important substitute, codonopsis. For each herb, I'll provide the following information:

- Common name, botanical name, and Chinese name
- Primary and secondary actions as a tonic (*chi*, blood, yang, and yin). See Chapter 12 for a more detailed explanation of these.
- Organs affected. Refer to Table 5.1 for a general description of the organs, and to the box in Chapter 12 for the symptoms of deficiency that may manifest in the major organs.
- Temperature. This refers to the warming, cooling, or neutral properties of the herb.

• Contraindications. Most of these are related to the temperature of the herb or to its digestibility. Warm herbs are contraindicated when heat signs are present, and cooling when cold signs predominate. (Refer to Table 4.2 for more details about signs of heat and cold.) The contraindications named refer to the use of the herb alone. Sometimes the contraindications can be overcome by including other herbs in a formula to balance the overall effect. This is a common practice in traditional Chinese formulas, but proceed with caution if you are self-prescribing herbs. Be on the lookout for signs of worsening of your condition that might come from taking a contraindicated herb, and stop taking it promptly if they appear. Please refer to my comments on self-medication in the Introduction.

• Dose. Dosages are given in grams. This may be confusing, because most herbs are sold by the ounce or pound, and most people do not have gram scales available. A postage or diet scale is usually in ounce gradations. The doses are for daily use, so if you are taking herbs twice a day, cut the dose in half. If you are self-prescribing tonic herbs, use the minimum doses. If you are making a formula of several herbs, include the normal dose for each herb, rather than reducing the dose because it is in a formula. A typical total dose of combined Chinese herbs for making teas can be several ounces. For eleuthero root, the dose of tincture is in milliliters. There are eight milliliters in a one-ounce bottle of tincture, the size usually available in health food stores.

• Products. At the end of the listings, I sometimes mention company products that include the herb. Please don't take these as exclusive endorsements. Many excellent tonic products are available, and it is beyond the scope of this book to describe them all. I provide information on where to order the products in Appendix A.

Common name: Asian ginseng, Chinese ginseng,
   Korean ginseng
Botanical name: *Panax ginseng*
Chinese name: *ren shen*
Primary action: *chi* tonic
Secondary actions: yin and blood tonic, sedative
Organs affected: Spleen, Lung, Heart
Temperature: slightly warm
Contraindications: heat signs, high blood pressure
Dose: 1–9 grams
Note: processed red ginseng is more heating, and is a yang
   tonic rather than a yin tonic.

I covered the Chinese use of ginseng in detail in Chapter 6. This is the most versatile and highly valued of the tonic family. It is unparalleled as a tonic to the overall *chi*; it strengthens the *chi*- and blood-building organs (Spleen and Lung), and also benefits the yin. Ginseng is calming to the Heart, which in the Chinese system is responsible for such symptoms as anxiety, palpitations, insomnia, excessive dreaming, and mental unrest.

Ginseng is available as whole roots in Chinese stores or by mail order. See the chapters in Section V on grades of ginseng and how to buy them.

In China, a common way to take whole roots is to make a tea or alcohol extract along with jujube dates. I'll provide details of how to do this in Chapter 15. Some possible combinations are:

   ginseng and jujube dates
   ginseng and astragalus
   ginseng with atractylodes, poria, and licorice

A wide variety of ginseng products — powders, tablets, capsules, liquid extracts, and teas — is available in health food stores, drug stores, and supermarkets. Their quality is highly variable (see "ginseng scams" in Chapter 17). A common Chinese liquid product called Ginseng Extractum is available in Chinese stores or through East Earth Tradewinds.

Another common product in China, often available in health food stores in the U.S., is *Ren Shen Feng Wang Jiang*. Sometimes the name is run together: *Renshenfengwangjiang*. This is a combination of ginseng and royal jelly, in liquid form, packaged in small vials. If you can't find it in a store, you can order it by the Chinese name from East Earth Tradewinds, or as Ginseng/Royal Jelly from the Institute for Traditional Medicine. K'an Herbals carries the Plum Flower brand from China, made with high-grade herbs and containing no chemical preservatives or sugars, under the name Imperial Ginseng and Royal Jelly.

The American companies listed in Appendix A all make ginseng products that are generally superior to Chinese products, because they use higher-grade starting material. Some excellent products are listed in the following pages.

Jade Chinese Herbals

These products are made by one of the most reputable companies in the Chinese herb business. Their product called Heavenly Ginsengs contains the highest grades of ginseng available, including a tiny amount of genuine wild Chinese ginseng, which can cost tens of thousands of dollars per root. It also includes *yi-sun* ginseng, a cultivated variety that closely resembles wild ginseng. Their Nine Ginsengs combines good-quality shiu chu and red kirin ginseng with tienchi ginseng and other tonic herbs in the "seng" family. They also make a simple ginseng extract.

Dragon Eggs

This product line includes a number of tonic herb formulas and single herbs. Four Ginsengs, Sage's Ginseng, and Shiu Chu/Kirin Ginseng are all made from superior grades of ginseng. If you can't find these in stores, they are available through East Earth Tradewinds.

Other Brands

High quality concentrated ginseng extracts are also available from Gaia Herbs, HerbPharm, and McZand Herbals.

Common name: American ginseng
Botanical name: *Panax quinquefolium*
Chinese name: *xi yang shen*
Primary action: yin tonic
Secondary action: mild *chi* tonic
Organs affected: Lung, Stomach, Kidney
Temperature: cool
Contraindications: cold signs with abdominal bloating
Dose: 3–9 grams

I covered the Chinese use of American ginseng in detail in Chapter 6. I recommend that you don't think of it as a substitute for or equivalent of Asian ginseng, but take it on its own indications. Other herbs, such as codonopsis or prince ginseng, are better substitutes for Asian ginseng. If you take Asian ginseng regularly, you might consider switching to American ginseng during hot weather the way some Chinese do. Asian ginseng is contraindicated when you are hot and sweating, but American ginseng is perfect for this.

Think of American ginseng as ginseng for people who are deficient and hot, with a racing pulse. It can help cool, calm, moisten, and strengthen a run-down system. It is well suited to stressed, overworked, and overactive Americans who have injured their yin function. Because it specifically strengthens the lungs, it would be a valuable addition to a formula to build athletic endurance, especially for sports played in hot weather.

Herbalist and acupuncturist Michael Tierra suggests that American ginseng is a better overall tonic for stressed-out Americans than is Asian ginseng, which can create tension and nervousness. American ginseng is calming rather than stimulating. "If you ask the proprietor of a Chinese herb store which ginseng is the better tonic, they will tell you Asian ginseng," says Tierra. "If you ask them what kind *they* are taking, they will often name American ginseng." Tierra also suggests that American ginseng is better for patients with AIDS or diabetes, who often have yin deficiency with heat signs and lung problems; these match the indications for American ginseng.

American ginseng roots are available in Chinese stores or by mail order from White Crane, East Earth Tradewinds, Frontier Herbs, or Spring Wind. See Chapter 18 for a discussion of quality and how to buy them. American ginseng products are widely available as liquid extracts in health food stores or through the mail. HerbPharm and Gaia Herbs produce some excellent concentrated products. Use American ginseng in any formula that calls for both a mild *chi* tonic and a yin tonic. Some possible combinations are:

> American ginseng with jujube dates and lycium berries
> American ginseng with *he shou wu*
> American ginseng with licorice

Common names: Deer Antler, Cornu Cervi parvum
Chinese name: *lu rong*
Primary action: yang tonic
Secondary action: *chi* and blood tonic
Organs affected: Liver, Kidney
Temperature: warming
Contraindications: heat signs
Dose: 1–2 grams as powder; 3–5 grams cooked in a double boiler or per ounce of liquor if soaked in wine (Wine dose: 1 ounce).

Deer antler is one of many animal substances that Chinese herbalists use. I remember my instant curiosity and amazement the first time I saw a jar of scorpions next to jars of small dried lizards and seahorses on a Chinese herbalist's shelf. Although reminiscent of the stories of witches' brews, these seemingly strange substances have potent medicinal properties, containing hormones, secretions, and chemicals from the animals involved. The deer shed their antlers seasonally, and the discarded antlers are collected on the forest floor.

Deer antler is one of the premier tonics in Chinese medicine, where it has as great a reputation as ginseng's. It appeared in the *Divine Husbandman's Classic* in the first century A.D. Its reputation as a yang tonic is built around its power to restore sexual potency, but it is also used as a general tonic. It improves the appetite, deepens sleep, decreases fatigue, and improves work capacity. It is sometimes prescribed for failure to thrive in children. Because it is warming, it is not taken when heat signs predominate. Some possible combinations:

> antler with ginseng or codonopsis
> antler with ginseng, *dong quai*, and lycium
> antler with rehmannia and/or *dong quai*

Antler comes in thin slices. It is available in Chinese herb shops, or by mail order from sources in Appendix B. It can be boiled to make a tea. A common method used in China is to soak it in wine for a few weeks.

A Chinese antler extract called Pantocrin, and a potent American tonic called Antler/Athletic by Jade Chinese Herbals, are also available from the same sources. Antler/Athletic includes many other tonic herbs. Seven Forests brand, available from Health Concerns or the Institute for Traditional Medicine, also sells a product called Antler 8, which adds other herbs to deer antler to prevent overstimulation.

Common name: Asparagus root
Botanical names: *Asparagus cochinchinensis, racemosus, officinalis*
Chinese name: *tian men dong*
Primary action: yin tonic
Organs affected: Lung, Kidney
Temperature: cold
Contraindications: cold conditions
Dose: 6–15 grams

This member of the lily family is a major herb for treating signs of deficiency heat. It is soothing and moistening to dry and inflamed mucous membranes of the mouth, throat, and lungs. It has a sweet flavor and a chewy texture. It may be eaten alone; break off pieces of one root and eat it throughout the course of a day. Some possible combinations:

> asparagus with rehmannia and ginseng
> asparagus with American ginseng
> asparagus with lycium berries and red dates

Common name: Astragalus
Botanical name: *Astragalus membranaceus*
Chinese name: *huang chi*
Primary action: *chi* tonic, blood tonic
Organs affected: Lung, Spleen
Temperature: warm
Contraindications: heat signs
Dose: 9–30 grams

Astragalus, which appeared in the earliest book of Chinese medicine, is rapidly gaining fame in the West as an immune stimulant. To pigeonhole it as an immune herb, however, is to overlook its broader use as a tonic. It strengthens the system, especially the lungs, improves the digestion, and builds up the blood. It increases endurance and body weight in animals. Astragalus is also a significant diuretic. American varieties of astragalus are known as "locoweed" because of their overstimulating effects on cattle that eat too much of them.

In Chapter 2, I explained that some of the functions of *chi* are to protect the body against external changes in temperature, to control sweating, and to maintain the immune system. Collectively called "protective *chi*" (*wei chi* in Chinese), this function is like the shield around the Starship Enterprise on *Star Trek*. When overall *chi* becomes depleted, this protective *chi* is weakened, and we become more susceptible to colds and we sweat more easily. A deficiency of protective *chi* is what makes AIDS patients so susceptible to opportunistic infections, and astragalus has a demonstrated effect in strengthening AIDS patients. When a long-distance runner finishes a race with heat exhaustion, he or she has depleted *chi* to the point of losing regulation of sweating, and will lose fluid profusely. Astragalus is like Scotty in the engine room, working feverishly to restore overall power, and then circulating it to the shield before the Klingons can destroy the ship.

Astragalus, in combination with another tonic herb, ligustrum, gained fame in scientific circles in the 1980s as a possible immune-stimulating and anti-cancer herb. In one trial with 19 cancer patients, water extracts of astragalus restored the function of the T-cells in 90% of the patients. T-cells are the main immune cells that attack tumors. In another trial, these two herbs in a broader formula increased the survival time of cancer patients receiving chemotherapy. Unfortunately, funding for this promising research in the U.S. was dropped because any eventual product was not patentable, and a drug company would not be able to recoup its investment. Formulas based on these two herbs are used today in AIDS clinics at the Institute for Traditional Medicine in Portland, Oregon, and at the Qwan Yin Clinic in San Francisco.

A similar commercial formula, called Astra-8, is produced by the Health Concerns company in Oakland, California. When I attended the National College of Naturopathic Medicine in Portland, Oregon, Astra-8 formula was routinely given to AIDS patients in our clinic. A related product, Astraisatis, was later used in the Healing AIDS Research Project at Bastyr University in Seattle, Washington. That study, conducted on early-stage AIDS patients, showed that a combination of natural therapies helped delay the progression of AIDS.

The herbs contained in Astra-8 are:

astragalus	(*chi* tonic)
ligustrum	(yin tonic)
ganoderma	(*chi* and blood tonic)
eleuthero root	(*chi* tonic)
codonopsis	(*chi* tonic)
schizandra	(yin and yang tonic, restrains sweating)
licorice	(*chi* tonic, adjuvant)
oryza	(astringent, restrains sweating)
malt sugar	(*chi* tonic)

As a general tonic, herbalist Ron Teeguarden suggests that astragalus is superior to ginseng for people under 40. It is also beneficial for people who work or play outdoors for long periods of time and are exposed to cold wind. It has no known toxicity, but can cause discomfort if you take it alone when you have heat signs. I did so on several occasions before I learned my lesson. Each time, I soon felt ill at ease. A mild rash broke out on my legs, and my eyes got red and began to itch. I'm sure that, if I were a cow and I had taken much more of it, I would have bellowed and started a stampede. The commercial formulas I mention here contain balancing herbs to reduce this possible effect.

Astragalus is available as a long, yellow-colored, sliced root in Chinese stores or by mail order from the bulk herb sources in Appendix A. Simmer the root for about a half an hour to make a tea.

Because its main benefits are to the protective *chi*, astragalus is often combined with another more general *chi* tonic in formulas. Some possible combinations:

astragalus with ginseng
astragalus with atractylodes
astragalus with angelica
astragalus with *he shou wu* and licorice

Astragalus is also widely available in health food stores as encapsulated powders, teas, and tinctures. A Chinese pure astragalus product called Extractum Astragali is available in Chinese stores or by mail from East Earth Tradewinds. An excellent astragalus formula is Shield *Chi*, made by Jade Chinese Herbals.

The Ginseng and Astragalus formula from McZand Herbals is available in health food stores or by mail order.

Common name: Atractylodes
Botanical name: *Atractylodes macrocephala*
Chinese name: *bai zhu*
Primary action: *chi* tonic
Organs affected: Spleen, Stomach
Temperature: warm
Contraindications: heat signs
Dose: 4–9 grams

This herb has a reputation as the best of the tonics for Spleen *chi*. While many tonics benefit the Spleen function, atractylodes is most appropriate when such symptoms as diarrhea, vomiting, and lack of appetite accompany fatigue. It is an excellent overall tonic, increasing the body weight and improving endurance, and restraining excessive sweating. Atractylodes is a diuretic, and is used in China for edema (swelling) that accompanies Spleen *chi* deficiency. Atractylodes is one of the herbs in the Four Gentlemen formula, the most famous *chi* tonic formula in Chinese medicine (See Ginseng in Chapter 6). Chinese herbalist Ron Teeguarden says that atractylodes is an important herb for use in a weight-loss program. Its benefits in weight loss are due to normalization of the appetite and loss of water weight through its diuretic effects.

Atractylodes macrocephala (bai zhu) should not be confused with *Atractylodes lancea (cang zhu)*, which has many opposite effects. The latter herb is contraindicated in *chi* deficiency with excessive sweating, a condition that *atractylodes macrocephala* is used to treat.

Atractylodes is available in bulk in Chinese stores or by mail order. It is found as an ingredient in many commercial tonic formulas. Some possible combinations:

atractylodes and orange peel
atractylodes and licorice

Common name: Codonopsis
Botanical name: *Codonopsis pilosula*
Chinese name: *dang shen*
Primary effect: *chi* tonic
Secondary effect: yin tonic
Organs affected: Spleen, Lung
Temperature: neutral or slightly warm

Contraindications: none noted in Chinese literature
Dosage: 3–9 grams

Codonopsis is so similar to Chinese ginseng in its action that it is substituted for the more expensive ginseng in most formulas in medical practice in China today. Its price is about a tenth that of ginseng. It is not as strong or long-lasting in its effects as ginseng, and a double-sized dose of codonopsis replaces ginseng in formulas. The only situation where it is not substituted is in cases of serious life-threatening shock or other severe illness. According to Dan Bensky, who holds both Chinese and osteopathic medical degrees, and who co-authored the two most famous Chinese herbal reference texts in the U.S. (see the Bibliography), codonopsis is even considered superior to ginseng as a tonic to Spleen and Lung function. Codonopsis is not in the same botanical family as ginseng, but like ginseng, eleuthero root, and several other tonics, it contains saponin constituents. It is safer for general use than ginseng, because it does not have the tendency to generate heat with long-term use.

Codonopsis is superior to American ginseng as a substitute for Asian ginseng. Codonopsis is much cheaper than American ginseng, which is even more expensive than Asian ginseng. Its superiority is clear from the history of Oriental medicine. Both codonopsis and American ginseng were introduced into Chinese medical practice during the eighteenth century—codonopsis through discovery at home, and American ginseng through export. The Chinese were at first excited about American ginseng because it looks so much like their native variety. It was soon found to have very different properties, however, and was quickly assigned its own separate place in the Chinese *materia medica*. Codonopsis, on the other hand, quickly became a ginseng substitute,

TABLE 13.1
COMPARISON BETWEEN GINSENG AND CODONOPSIS

Ginseng	Codonopsis
sweet, slightly bitter	sweet
warm	neutral or slightly warm
strengthens Spleen function	strengthens Spleen function
benefits *chi* through Lungs	benefits *chi* through Lungs
benefits yin, generates fluids	benefits yin, generates fluids
powerful tonic to *chi*	mild tonic to *chi*
builds the blood	builds the blood
strengthens Stomach	
benefits Heart *chi*	
sedative effect	

and is used today more frequently than the rarer Asian ginseng in medical practice. Like Asian ginseng, codonopsis has secondary blood-tonifying properties, and is often included in formulas for anemia.

Chinese research has shown that codonopsis has immune-stimulating properties. It also raises the metabolism, decreases respiratory rate, and increases red blood cell counts.

Codonopsis is never used alone in China. Combine it with other *chi* or blood tonics, or with warming adjuvant herbs. Some combinations are:

> codonopsis with atractylodes
> codonopsis with astragalus and jujube dates
> codonopsis with *dong quai* and licorice
> codonopsis with ginger

Codonopsis is a common ingredient in herbal soup mixes available at Chinese herb stores. I ask for "herbal soup" mix, or "chicken soup" mix. The mixes come in packages to be cooked along with a pot of chicken soup. I make them up when I am feeling temporarily depleted from stress, or when the seasons change and I am susceptible to catching a cold. I make either chicken soup or lamb stew. You can also make up your own from herbs purchased separately in Chinese stores or through mail order.

Soup Mix

codonopsis (or ginseng)	2 parts	1 ounce
astragalus	2 parts	1 ounce
dioscorea	2 parts	1 ounce
lycium	2 parts	1 ounce
cordyceps	1 part	½ ounce

Cook with chicken and/or vegetables in 2 quarts of water.

Common name: Cordyceps
Botanical name: *Cordyceps sinensis*
Chinese name: *dong chong zia cao*
Primary action: tonifies both yin and yang
Organs affected: Lung, Kidney
Temperature: neutral
Contraindicated: exterior conditions
Dose: 5–12 grams

This strange-looking medicinal substance is a fungus that grows from the carcasses of the larva of various insects. It looks like a short, spindly growth protruding from the body of a small dried caterpillar. As odd as it looks, this is an important tonic. One prominent Chinese herbalist of the sixteenth century stated that cordyceps was as effective as ginseng in building up a depleted system. The more commonly held view is that it is not a *chi* tonic like ginseng, but it is used when a formula calls for a yang or yin tonic for Kidney function. It also tonifies depleted immune function, and is especially good for recovery from debilitating illnesses or symptoms of premature aging. Because it tonifies both yin and yang, it is safer for long-term use than the warmer yang tonics.

In China, cordyceps is often cooked in meat stews or with roast duck. It's available in bulk from Chinese stores or by mail order. Use a dozen pieces in a pot of stew.

Common name: Dendrobium
Botanical name: *Dendrobium nobile*
Chinese name: *shi hu*
Primary effect: yin tonic for deficiency heat
Organs affected: Lung, Kidney
Temperature: cold
Contraindications: cold or neutral conditions; abdominal distension; heavily coated tongue
Dose: 6–12 grams

The stems and leaves of this Chinese orchid are famous in China, and appeared in the earliest book of Chinese medicine. It is the premier tonic herb for clearing deficiency heat with thirst and prolonged low-grade fever. It is also useful for stomachache and/or dry heaves when heat signs are present.

According to Chinese herbalist Ron Teeguarden, dendrobium is a favorite of the Taoists for building sexual energy or recovering from sexual excess. He suggests that it may be taken with licorice as a daily tea.

In extremely large doses, this herb has caused convulsions in animals.

Common name: Dioscorea
Botanical name: *Dioscorea opposita*
Chinese name: *shan yao*
Primary actions: *chi* tonic
Secondary action: balanced yin and yang tonic
Organs affected: Spleen, Lung, Kidney
Temperature: neutral
Contraindications: excess conditions
Dose: 9–30 grams

This *chi* tonic is most often used as a secondary herb to support other stronger tonics. Dioscorea is ubiquitous in tonic soup mixes (see codonopsis above). It is useful in any formula to treat weak digestion, weak lungs, debilitation due to stress, or weakened sexual function. Some combinations are:

> dioscorea with poria for weak digestion
> dioscorea with codonopsis for energy
> dioscorea with antler for Kidney deficiency

Common name: *Dong quai*
Botanical name: *Angelica sinensis*
Chinese names: *dang gui, tang kwei*
Primary action: Blood tonic
Secondary action: yin tonic
Organs affected: Heart, Liver, Spleen
Temperature: warm
Contraindications: heat signs, diarrhea, pregnancy
Dose: 3–15 grams

Dong quai is one of the most famous herbs in China, and possibly used more often than any other. It appeared in the oldest book of Chinese medicine, *The Divine Husbandman's Classic of the Materia Medica*. Dong quai benefits a wide variety of gynecological disorders, including painful, irregular, excessive, or scanty menstruation, vaginal infection, or infertility. It is really like two herbs in one, because it both builds the blood and promotes blood circulation through its warming effects. Because of these blood-circulating properties, it is sometimes used after painful trauma that causes bruising; the *dong quai* will help to heal the bruise. It is used the same way for the pain of arthritis. In Chinese medicine, pain is often considered a sign of either "stuck *chi*" or "congealed blood." Chinese research has shown that *dong quai* has both sedative and pain-relieving properties. Its warming, circulation-promoting properties make *dong quai* contraindicated when heat signs are present, especially deficiency heat, which it will aggravate.

According to legend, the Chinese name *dang qui* came from an unhappy love affair. A young, recently married man left for the mountains to prove his manhood after being taunted by other men in the village. He arranged with his wife that if he did not return in three years, she would be free to remarry. The three years passed but he did not return, and the wife reluctantly took a new husband. Soon the first husband returned, however, and both were heartbroken. Her health declined and she became weak. The former husband gave her the root of an unknown plant that he found in the mountains, and her health was restored. The Chinese characters *dang* and *gui* have three possible meanings when combined: "should come back," "missing the husband," and "proper order." "Proper order" fits the medicinal action of *dong quai*, which restores both the blood and its proper circulation. The image of the wife—weak, pale, and in poor overall health—fits the picture of the ideal *dong quai* patient.

Dong quai is readily available in bulk in any Chinese store or through mail order. It comes in large, acrid-smelling slices. It may be taken alone, in small coin-sized pieces, or brewed as a simple tea. Brew it in a container with a lid to keep in the volatile warming substances. Some possible combinations are:

> *dong quai* with astragalus
> *dong quai* with rehmannia
> *dong quai* with peony and lycium
> *dong quai* with jujube dates

Dong quai is part of the Four Things Decoction, the most famous women's tonic in China. The formula, which regulates the menstrual cycle, also includes equal parts of rehmannia, peony, and ligustrum.

A popular Chinese formula, readily available in stores or through mail order is *Tan Kwei Gin* (pronounced "geen"), a liquid containing about 70% *dong quai*, with the rest of the formula being balancing *chi* tonics and adjuvant herbs.

Common names: Eleuthero root, Siberian ginseng
Botanical names: *Eleutherococcus senticosus,*
   Acanthopanax senticosus
Chinese names: *ci-wu-jia, wu-jia-pi*
Primary use: *chi* tonic
Organs affected: Kidney
Temperature: warm
Contraindications: heat signs, insomnia
Dose: 5 grams to 1 ounce. Tincture 2–20 ml/day. Use lower
   doses in the sick or the elderly.

Eleutherococcus senticosus, or eleuthero root, seems to be a plant fated to be misnamed. It is sold widely in North

America as "Siberian ginseng," but it is not a ginseng at all. Scientists cannot agree on its Latin name, and its original Chinese name—*wu-jia-pi*—was shared with as many as 13 other plants, many of them with entirely different properties than eleuthero root. I'll discuss these naming problems in some detail, because eleuthero root is mistakenly thought by many consumers in the U.S. to be an equivalent of Chinese and Korean ginseng, and because the confusion in Chinese names may have led to toxicity in some American products.

Eleuthero is in the same botanical family as ginseng, but this does not mean that it is ginseng. The name "Siberian ginseng" was devised by marketers hoping to capitalize on the popularity of true ginseng. Scientists classify plants and animals according to family, genus, and species. A human being—*Homo sapiens*—belongs to the *Primate* family, the *Homo* genus, and the *sapiens* species within that genus. True ginsengs (of the *Panax* genus) are in the *Araliaceae* family. Chinese and American ginsengs are, respectively, the *ginseng* and *quinquefolium* species of *Panax*.

Eleutherococcus senticosus is also in the *Araliaceae* family, but is not in the *Panax* genus. To clarify the relationship, a modern human (*Homo sapiens*) and a prehistoric ancestor to the human (*Homo erectus*) would have important similarities, being in the same genus, and significant differences, being of different species. Others in the same *Primate* family but not in the *Homo* genus, including monkeys, chimpanzees, gorillas, baboons, and even tiny gibbons, are even less like humans. Botanically, *Eleutherococcus senticosus*, being in the same family as *Panax ginseng* or *Panax quinquefolium*, has some similarities to those plants, but the differences between them are as great as those between a human and a chimpanzee.

Refer to the list below to see eleuthero root's place in the Araliaceae family.

Scientists today do not even agree on the genus name *Eleutherococcus* for eleuthero root. Russian botanists gave it its first Latin botanical name, *Hedera senticosa*, in 1856. In 1859, the Russian botanist Maximowicz removed the plant from the *Hedera* genus, named it *Eleutherococcus senticosus*, and recognized *Eleutherococcus* as a distinct genus of its own. Later the same year, a German botanist combined the *Eleutherococcus* genus with the *Acanthopanax* genus, which formerly had been a subgenus of *Panax*, the genus of true ginsengs. Most botanists worldwide now call the genus *Eleutherococcus*, but Chinese scientists still call it *Acanthopanax*, and call eleuthero root *Acanthopanax senticosus*.

Ginseng's Botanical Cousins

Some tonic plants in the Araliaciae family:

Panax genus

Panax ginseng	Chinese or Korean ginseng
Panax quinquefolium	American ginseng
Panax japonicus	Japanese ginseng
Panax pseudoginseng	tienchi ginseng

Eleutherococcus (Acanthopanax) genus

Eleutherococcus senticosus	eleuthero, Siberian ginseng, *ci-wu-jia*, *wu-jia-pi*
Eleutherococcus gracilistylus	*wu-jia-pi*
Eleutherococcus sessiflorus	*wu-jia-pi*

Aralia genus

Aralia racemosa	American spikenard
Aralia californica	American spikenard
Aralia nudicaulis	American spikenard
Aralia quinquefolia	American spikenard

Oplopanax genus

Oplopanax horridum	Devil's club

The Mystery of *Wu-jia-pi*

The Chinese common name for eleuthero root is even more confusing than the Western Latin names. The *Divine Husbandman's Classic* from the first century B.C. listed a plant called *wu-jia-pi* as useful for promoting energy and for curing rheumatism. It was classified in the middle category of medicines, not as a tonic. Which plant the *Classic* refers to is not clear, because at least 13 different plants, probably including *Eleutherococcus (Acanthopanax) senticosus*, *Eleutherococcus (Acanthopanax) gracilistylus*, and *Periploca sepium*, were used in China over the centuries, and all were called *wu-jia* or *wu-jia-pi*.

A Chinese physician in about 500 A.D. commented that "the better *wu-jia-pi* is the five-leaved one"—probably *Eleutherococcus senticosus*, which usually has five leaves. Later, in the sixteenth century, Chinese physician Li Shih-Chen repeated that the "five-leafed" *wu-jia* was the better one, and drew a picture of it, which closely resembles *Eleutherococcus senticosus*. He furthermore upgraded the classification of the herb from the middle class of herbs to the highest class—the tonics. Note that, traditionally, the root bark of *wu-jia-pi* plants was often used in Chinese medicine, instead of the whole root.

TABLE 13.2
CHINESE PLANTS HISTORICALLY COMING
UNDER THE CLASSICAL NAME *WU-JIA-PI*

Latin Name	Modern Chinese Name
Eleutherococcus (Acanthopanax) *senticosus*	ci-wu-jia
Eleutherococcus (Acanthopanax) *gracilistylus*	wu-jia-pi
Periploca sepium	xiang-jian-pi

In recent decades, the Chinese have renamed the three species that commonly fall under the name *wu-jia-pi*. *Eleutherococcus senticosus* is now called *ci-wu-jia*, and the whole root is specified; *Eleutherococcus gracilistylus* (root bark) is now the only plant that will be called *wu-jia-pi*; and *Periploca sepium* (root bark) is now called *xiang-jian-pi*.

This confusion of the three plants called *wu-jia-pi* may have had a negative effect on the reputation of eleuthero in China. The three were apparently used interchangeably, but the last of the species, *Periploca sepium*, has the potential of being toxic, and cannot be taken for long periods. It is possible that this plant, and the weaker effects of the less-powerful *Eleutherococcus gracilistylus*, gave *Eleutherococcus senticosus* a bad name; this may be one reason why eleuthero is not more widely used today in China. Substitution of periploca for eleuthero root has caused toxic reactions from products labeled as Siberian ginseng in the U.S. See the discussion on product adulteration in Chapter 17. Another thing that may have hurt its reputation is that only its root bark was traditionally used. It took Russian researchers in the 1950s to discover the more powerful tonic properties of the whole root.

Eleuthero and *Chi* in Chinese Medicine

Eleuthero has never held a place in Chinese medicine comparable to that of Asian or American ginseng, and this reflects its weaker activity as a tonic. It is recognized as a tonic for Kidney *chi*, aiding in stress resistance and sexual restoration, but it is not used like ginseng, nor is it ever substituted for ginseng in China. Even after the physician Li Shih-Chen clarified the botanical identification of eleuthero and upgraded its status to that of the tonic herbs nearly 400 years ago, it never caught on as a general *chi* tonic. As a comparison, consider that when the Chinese came into contact with American ginseng in the 1700s, a tremendous trade for it developed that continues today, even though it is not as powerful a tonic as Asian ginseng. Codonopsis also entered Chinese medicine in the 1700s, and it quickly became a ginseng substitute.

After Russian researchers claimed, 40 years ago, that eleuthero root is a more powerful tonic than Chinese ginseng, Chinese scientists took an interest in it and entered it in the official Chinese pharmacopoeia as a tonic and adaptogen. But no trade comparable to that of American ginseng has ever developed. The Chinese still pay top dollar for good Chinese and American ginseng, which are rare in the wild and must be cultivated at great expense, even though eleuthero grows widely as a common weed. To use baseball terminology, if ginseng is "major league," and American ginseng is "minor league," eleutherococcus is "college ball." It may still be a ball game, but while the majors and minors are around, baseball lovers aren't likely to flock to a college ball game on Saturday afternoon. Eleuthero bark is still prepared in rice wine and used, not as a tonic, but to treat arthritis. Eleuthero root is used today in some Chinese hospitals along with chemo-therapy in order to reduce the toxic side effects of the cancer treatment.

A tremendous amount of research into the adaptogenic effects of eleuthero root was done in the former Soviet Union. It is widely used today in Russia as an adaptogen to increase resistance to stress, colds, and flu, and is very effective for those purposes. The Russian product is extracted in 33% alcohol. Eleuthero root has more immediate stimulating effects than most of the tonic herbs, and this may contribute to the misconception that it is a superior tonic. It can also easily overstimulate, with symptoms such as insomnia, anxiety, and tension in the shoulders.

Eleuthero root, usually labeled Siberian Ginseng, is available in bulk, capsules, or tinctures in most health food stores and herb shops. It would be wise to choose the tinctures, because the great volume of research into eleuthero root was performed on alcohol extracts. The HerbPharm company makes a product according to the specifications of the Russian research, then concentrates it to double strength.

Common name: Eucommia
Botanical name: *Eucommia ulmoides*
Chinese name: *ðu zhong*
Primary action: yang tonic
Organs affected: Kidney, Liver
Temperature: warm
Contraindications: heat signs
Dose: 6–15 grams

Eucommia is used as a yang tonic to treat sexual weakness and to strengthen the bones. It also aids in the smooth flow of *chi* and blood, and is sometimes used as an adjuvant in tonic formulas to ensure circulation. In its own right, eucommia tea has been found to have blood-pressure-lowering properties and anti-inflammatory effects. Eucommia is used in China to prevent miscarriage.

Eucommia is available in bulk in Chinese stores and through mail order. It can be used alone as a tea for mildly elevated blood pressure. Most often it is not used alone, but is added to other yang tonic formulas to promote circulation.

Common name: *Fo-Ti*
Botanical name: *Polygonum multiflorum*
Chinese name: *he shou wu*
Primary actions: blood and yin tonic
Organs affected: Kidney, Liver
Temperature: slightly warm
Contraindications: Spleen deficiency, excess mucous
Dose: 9 grams–1 ounce

He shou wu is one of the most famous tonics in China, used as a general tonic to postpone or reverse the effects of aging. It is named after a man in seventh-century China named He. A retired farmer, too old to work the land any more, he had to go to the forest to search for food during a famine. He returned several months later, and the villagers noticed that his grey hair had begun to turn black, and that he appeared to be younger than when he left. He explained that he had been forced to eat the roots of a particular plant, which the people named in his honor. *He shou wu* means "Black-haired Mr. He." The herb first appeared in an official Chinese medical text in 713 A.D. *Fo-Ti*, the common name in the U.S., was invented by marketing concerns in the U.S. in the 1970s.

The power of this herb is demonstrated by its popularity in Japan, where it is called *kashuu*. It was first introduced there in the early 1700s. Its use spread rapidly, and it remains today one of the most popular tonic herbs there. This is one of my personal favorites as a tonic herb. I once used it with some other herbs to quickly restore me from a state of extreme exhaustion (see my story in Chapter 2) and I still use it from time to time when I become run down from overwork, especially working late at night. It is used in traditional Chinese medicine for deficient blood and yin syndromes with symptoms such as insomnia, dizziness, or blurred vision. It is also used for deficient Kidney syndromes, such as premature grey hair, weak lower back or knees, premature ejaculation, and infertility.

Although *he shou wu* is slightly warming, it is not contraindicated in conditions that are usually considered hot. In fact, it will even decrease a fever. In clinical trials, *he shou wu* tea and glycyrrhiza were given to 17 patients with the recurring fever of malaria. In 15 cases, the symptoms disappeared completely; the two recurrences were successfully treated with the same formula. *He shou wu* has sedative and blood pressure-lowering properties. It is used by both conventional and traditional Chinese physicians to lower cholesterol. In a clinical trial, a simple tea of *he shou wu* was given to 88 patients with high cholesterol. Cholesterol levels decreased in 78 patients, and increased in 8 (the increase was not necessarily due to the *he shou wu*). In animal experiments, *he shou wu* increased red blood cell count and enhanced resistance to cold.

"Black-haired Mr. He" comes either raw or processed. The processed form is the one available in the U.S. The roots are cooked in the broth of black beans, and acquire the deep-brown color of the beans. The unprocessed roots have a laxative property that the processing mostly removes. In China, herbalists use the unprocessed root as a laxative and to detoxify boils and similar accumulations. Side effects of the processed root can include increased frequency of the stool, mild abdominal pain, or a flushed face. These will usually pass in a day or two.

The roots are available in any Chinese store, or through mail order. *He shou wu* and ginseng, combined in equal parts, makes a superb general tonic. Prepare them as a tea or wine extraction (see Chapter 15 for details). Chinese texts caution against cooking *he shou wu* in a metal container. Some other possible combinations:

he shou wu with codonopsis
he shou wu with *dong quai*
he shou wu with eucommia
he shou wu with peony and ligusticum

Two popular and inexpensive Chinese products available in Chinese stores or through East Earth Tradewinds are *Shou Wu Pian* and *Shou Wu Chih*. The first is 100% *he shou wu* with sugar. The second, a liquid, combines *he shou wu* with *dong quai* and some other herbs. Fo-Ti Dragon Eggs, an American product, is more expensive but is much more potent.

Common name: Ganoderma
Botanical name: *Ganoderma lucidum*
Chinese name: *ling zhi*
Properties: *chi* tonic
Organs affected: All five major organs, depending on type
Temperature: warm

Contraindications: signs of excess
Dose: 3–9 grams

The ganoderma mushroom, sometimes called by the Japanese name *reishi* in the U.S., is an immune-stimulating sedative. It first appeared in the oldest book of Chinese medicine. This book identified six types of *ling zhi* by their colors: red, black, blue, yellow, white, and purple. They are all *chi* tonics, but each one affects different organ systems. Although all are called *ling zhi*, some of these are actually different species in the *ganoderma* genus. The two types commonly found in the U.S. are red and black. They look nothing alike, the red being more round and compact, and the black being larger and more fibrous or fleshy. The red tastes bitter, and the black more salty. The red *ling zhi* affects the *chi* and all the organs; it especially affects the Heart with sedative and calming properties. The black has a stronger effect on the Kidney.

A large amount of scientific research has been conducted into ganoderma, especially in Japan. It is an immune-stimulant, building resistance to infection and tumors. It also has cardiotonic properties, lowering serum cholesterol and increasing blood circulation through the coronary arteries. A number of clinical trials have shown it to be effective for chronic bronchitis.

Ganoderma is especially useful as a sedative for the nervousness, restlessness, and insomnia that often accompany general deficiency.

Go into any Chinese store and ask for *ling zhi*, and the proprietor will show you several products to choose from. The one I like claims to combine all six types of ganoderma. You can also buy the mushrooms in bulk through the mail from sources listed in Appendix B, and make them into a tea.

Ganoderma is a common ingredient in tonic formulas, usually added for its immune-stimulating and sedative actions.

Common name: Glehnia
Botanical name: *Glehnia littoralis*
Chinese name: *bei sha shen*
Primary action: yin tonic, Lung tonic
Organs affected: Lung, Stomach
Temperature: cool
Contraindications: acute cough or cold signs
Dose: 9–15 grams

This herb is included in yin tonic formulas when a dry, chronic cough is a predominant symptom. It is also used for dry, itchy skin. Research in China shows that it has an analgesic effect and can reduce fevers.

Glehnia is available in bulk in Chinese stores or through mail order. It may be added to other formulas for deficient yin.

Common name: Jujube dates, red dates
Botanical name: *Zizyphus jujuba*
Chinese names: *da zao, hong zao*
Primary action: *chi* tonic
Secondary actions: yin tonic, sedative, adjuvant to harmonize harsh herbs
Organs affected: Spleen, Stomach, Heart
Temperature: neutral
Contraindications: abdominal bloating and distension; intestinal parasites
Dose: 3–10 dates

Red dates are a common ingredient in many tonic formulas. These pleasant-tasting fruits are a *chi* and Spleen tonic in their own right, but are included in formulas as adjuvants to enhance digestion and absorption. Red dates are a natural counterpart to warming *chi* tonics like ginseng or astragalus, and are of benefit in any yang tonic formula. They also moisten a dried-out system, and have a sedative effect. Red dates will be useful in any tonic formula for insomnia. Animal research shows that they will increase weight and endurance, and may have a healing and protective effect on the liver.

Red dates are available in any Chinese store or through mail order. Fresh dates are usually available in Chinese stores, and are of higher quality than dried dates. They can be eaten alone as snacks, or cooked with foods. When my digestion is feeling a little sluggish, I like to chew on one or two dates. In China, ginseng is usually taken as a tea or alcohol prepared with jujube dates to improve its digestibility.

Common name: Licorice root
Botanical names: *Glycyrrhiza uralensis, Glycyrrhiza glabra*
Chinese name: *gan cao*
Primary action: *chi* tonic
Organs affected: Primarily Spleen and Lung; all 12 organs to some extent
Temperature: neutral (honey-fried licorice is warming)
Contraindications: nausea, heart disease, kidney disease, high blood pressure, pregnancy, edema (honey-fried licorice: heat signs)
Dose: 3–12 grams

Licorice is famous in the West as a candy, but most licorice candy is made from anise flavorings rather than from real licorice. This herb, which was placed in the superior class of herbs in the oldest book of Chinese medicine, is used more than any other herb in Chinese formulas. It is probably the most versatile herb in either Eastern or Western pharmacopoeias, and can relieve respiratory illnesses, digestive problems, menstrual disorders, inflammatory conditions, auto-immune diseases, and chronic liver disease. In Chinese medicine, licorice root is said to affect all the meridians and organ systems, and this is its value in a tonic formula; it can guide the *chi* into all the systems. It also moderates the side effects of strong herbs.

Research has shown that licorice by itself can treat a wide variety of diseases:

- It strengthens the digestion, and has cleared ulcers in 80% of patients in clinical trials.
- It is an expectorant for the lungs, and research shows that it is as effective as codeine as a cough suppressant.
- It has a mild estrogenic effect, and is used in many Western gynecological formulas.
- Glycyrrhizin, the principal active constituent of licorice, is used by conventional physicians in Japan to treat chronic hepatitis. In Chinese clinical trials, licorice cleared up 70% of cases of chronic hepatitis after two to three months of treatment.
- In AIDS patients, it can restore normal liver function.
- It has anti-allergy effects similar to cortisone, although not as strong. When taken with cortisone, it increases its effect and duration.
- It can be of benefit in treating bronchial asthma.

Licorice root can cause side effects when taken in large doses and for long periods. It stimulates the adrenal glands and adds to the effect of steroid hormones, causing high blood pressure, edema, headache, and loss of potassium.

These effects were first observed in people who ate large amounts of concentrated licorice extracts in candy. Later, they were observed in the long-term clinical use of licorice for the treatment of ulcers and hepatitis. These symptoms do not appear with normal use in tonic formulas.

Honey-fried licorice has somewhat different properties than raw licorice. It is more heating, and has stronger *chi*-tonic properties. It is not available this way commercially, but you can make it yourself. Warm a moderate amount of honey in a skillet until it turns a brownish color. Then add some water to moisten it and stir-fry the licorice in it until it has absorbed enough honey to turn a darker color.

I once experienced the heating effect of this form in a dramatic way. I was eating small pieces of American ginseng and honey-fried licorice while working on a grueling writing project. After four or five days, I developed heat signs: racing pulse, flushed face, and insomnia. I first thought that it was due to the American ginseng, but when I later took the ginseng without the licorice, no such signs appeared. I am prone to deficiency heat, and should have known better. During this same period I met a friend at a dance, and gave her a jar of honey-fried licorice as a present. She is also prone to deficiency heat, and was hot from dancing. She ate a piece of the licorice, and within five minutes felt so hot that she had to sit down.

Licorice is readily available in Chinese stores, health food stores, herb shops, or through the mail. I prefer the Chinese licorice because it comes in small angular slices that are easy to use, although Western forms are as effective. You can chew the Chinese slices like candy, which I do for a dry cough, and they are easy to honey-fry.

Licorice is a member of the famous Four Gentlemen tonic formula, which also includes codonopsis, atractylodes, and poria. It is a valuable addition to any tonic formula. Try a tea of ginseng and licorice in equal parts. A wonderful and very inexpensive tonic is equal parts of codonopsis and licorice.

Common name: Ligustrum, Privet
Botanical name: *Ligustrum lucidum*
Chinese name: *nu zhen zi*
Primary use: yin tonic
Organs affected: Liver, Kidney
Temperature: neutral
Contraindications: deficient yang; diarrhea with cold signs
Dose: 5–15 grams

This herb is not used alone, but is included in formulas for deficient yin when Kidney deficiency is predominant (symptoms might include premature grey hair, dizziness, blurry vision, low back pain, weak legs and knees, and tinnitus).

Ligustrum has received attention in Western research as part of a formula with astragalus. Astragalus-ligustrum combinations have been used successfully to treat cancer and AIDS. See the discussion under astragalus.

Ligustrum is rarely available in health food stores, but can be found in Chinese stores or by mail order.

Common name: Lycium berries
Botanical name: *Lycium chinensis*
Chinese name: *gao chi zhi*
Primary use: blood and yin tonic

Organs affected: Liver, Kidney
Temperature: neutral
Contraindications: abdominal bloating, inflammatory
  conditions
Dose: 6–15 grams

These fruits, which resemble small red currants, are common in Chinese herb formulas. Besides nourishing the blood and yin, they are useful for Kidney deficiency, with such symptoms as lower back pain, weak knees, sexual weakness, dizziness, and blurred vision. They are also used in Chinese hospitals to treat high blood pressure.

They are available in Chinese stores or through East Earth Tradewinds. Some possible combinations:

lycium and ginseng
lycium and codonopsis
lycium and rehmannia
lycium and schizandra

They may also be nibbled as snacks or used in cooking. I like to put a handful on top of a pot of just-cooked basmati rice. Cover and let them steam for a while. Then stir them in. This makes a delicious, colorful, health-building rice dish.

Common name: Morindae
Botanical name: *Morinda officinalis*
Chinese name: *ba ji tian*
Primary action: yang tonic
Organs affected: Liver, Kidney
Temperature: warm
Contraindication: deficiency heat
Dose: 5–15 grams

Although this herb appeared in the oldest book of Chinese medicine, it is not used alone. It is included in yang and blood tonic formulas when cold signs are present and Kidney symptoms predominate. It strengthens the muscles and bones. You'll find it in Chinese stores or by mail order from the sources listed in Appendix B. It combines well with eucommia, *dong quai*, rehmannia, or lycium.

Common name: Peony
Botanical name: *Paeonia lactiflora*
Chinese name: *bai shao*
Primary action: blood and yin tonic
Organs affected: Liver, Spleen
Temperature: cold
Contraindications: diarrhea with cold signs
Dose: 6–15 grams

Peony root is an important women's tonic in Chinese medicine. It is closely related medicinally to asparagus root. While having entirely different textures, they both have significant amounts of the same constituent, *asparagine*. This is a primary tonic herb for menstrual cramps and other menstrual disorders. It is often used in place of *dong quai*, which is warming, when heat signs are present. It has antispasmodic properties which help all kinds of cramps and spasms. It is a valuable addition to *chi* tonic formulas, which can cause tension, because it relieves the tension. It is also used to relieve night sweats in patients who have deficient yin. Chinese research shows that it lowers blood pressure.

Peony is one of the members of the Four Things Decoction, the most famous women's tonic in China, which also includes *dong quai*, rehmannia, and ligusticum.

It is available in bulk in Chinese stores and by mail order from sources listed in Appendix B. Some possible combinations:

> peony with licorice
> peony with *dong quai*
> peony with rehmannia

Common name: Poria
Botanical name: *Poria cocos*
Chinese name: *fu ling*
Primary action: *chi* tonic, especially Spleen *chi*; sedative
Organs affected: Spleen, Heart, Lung
Temperature: neutral
Contraindications: frequent urination with cold signs
Dose: 9–15 grams

This plant is a white, round fungus that grows underground on the roots of conifer trees. It was known in turn-of-the-century Western herbalism as "tuckahoe," named for the hoe that is necessary to dig it up from the tree roots. The main action of poria is on the Spleen. It drains accumulated moisture in the upper digestive tract and relieves abdominal bloating. It is included in many *chi* or blood tonic formulas which can have a tendency to promote abdominal bloating. It is a strong diuretic and a first-class sedative, providing relief for insomnia and anxiety. Chinese research shows that it will lower blood pressure and blood sugar levels.

Poria is available in bulk in Chinese stores or through the mail from sources listed in Appendix B. It is a member of the famous Four Gentlemen tonic formula, which also includes ginseng (or codonopsis), atractylodes, and licorice.

Common name: Prince ginseng
Botanical name: *Pseudostellaria heterophylla*
Chinese names: *hai er shen, tai zi shen*
Primary action: *chi* tonic
Secondary action: yin tonic
Organs affected: Spleen, Lung, Heart
Temperature: neutral
Contraindications: none noted
Dose: 6–15 grams

Prince ginseng is not related to Chinese ginseng botanically, but its action is similar, although weaker. Prince ginseng roots look like tiny Chinese ginseng roots. Prince ginseng is milder than codonopsis, but is a worthy substitute for ginseng for people who find ginseng or codonopsis too stimulating. Prince ginseng in combination with schizandra was found effective in Chinese clinical trials for nervous exhaustion.

Prince ginseng is available in Chinese stores or by mail order. It costs about a tenth the price of ginseng. Use it like ginseng in a tea with jujube dates, or combine it with schizandra berries. Prince ginseng is sometimes used as a component in tonic formulas found in health food stores.

Common name: Rehmannia
Botanical name: *Rehmannia glutinosa*
Chinese names: *shi di huang, di huang*
Primary uses: blood and yin tonic
Organs affected: Liver, Kidney, Heart
Temperature: slightly warm
Contraindications: weak digestion, abdominal bloating, excess phlegm, pain from stuck *chi*
Dose: 9 grams to 28 grams (1 ounce)

Rehmannia appeared in the oldest book of Chinese medicine, and remains a famous women's tonic today. It is a primary herb in formulas to tonify blood and yin deficiency, with symptoms such as paleness, dizziness, palpitations, insomnia, and menstrual dysfunction. It is also the principal herb for treating deficient yin when Kidney symptoms are predominant, such as night sweats, lower back pain, infertility, sexual weakness, and slow healing of bones or flesh. It is especially important in treating wasting diseases, such as diabetes.

Rehmannia can lower blood pressure. In a Chinese clinical trial, 62 patients with high blood pressure and no contraindications for rehmannia took it for two weeks. Both blood pressure and serum cholesterol levels fell.

Rehmannia can be hard to digest, and overuse can lead to abdominal bloating and diarrhea. Initial side effects, such as mild diarrhea, abdominal pain, dizziness, or low energy, will usually disappear with continued use.

Rehmannia comes either as a raw root or in a prepared, steamed form. Both have the same tonic properties. The steamed roots are black and have warming properties, while the raw root is cooling and is sometimes preferred in China during hot weather. Prepared roots are most common in this country, but raw roots can be obtained by mail order from Frontier Herbs.

Rehmannia is one of the herbs in the Four Things Decoction, the most famous women's tonic in China. The other herbs are *dong quai*, peony, and ligusticum. Rehmannia combines well with *dong quai* or asparagus root as a simple tea.

One way to prepare rehmannia is to soak it in wine for three weeks. Add a little fennel seed or cardamom to promote digestion. Take doses of a wineglass-full a day. Wine itself is considered to promote circulation in Chinese medicine.

Rehmannia is a common ingredient in Chinese products. One popular formula is Women's Precious Pills, available in Chinese stores or through East Earth Tradewinds. K'an Herbals sells an excellent variation of this product, manufactured from high-quality herbs and using ginseng in place of the codonopsis in the original formula. Another Chinese product featuring rehmannia is *Chih Pai Di Huang Wan*, which also contains cooling herbs for the hot flashes of menopause.

Common name: Royal jelly
Chinese name: *feng wang jiang*
Principal use: *chi* and blood tonic
Organs affected: Liver and Spleen
Temperature: neutral
Contraindications: excess conditions

In a beehive, the worker bees produce a glandular secretion from honey known as *royal jelly*. This makes up the total diet of the queen bee of the hive. It must be a superb diet because the queen lives for five to six years, while the workers only live four to five months. Royal jelly, a *chi* and blood tonic, is not a traditional Chinese medicine, being only recently discovered. However, it is very popular in China, mixed with other tonics in the form of patent medicines.

These patents are a very common sight in North American health food stores. I already discussed *Ren Shen Feng Wang Jiang*, ginseng and royal jelly, under Asian ginseng. Other common products are *Ling Zhi Feng Wang Jiang*, ganoderma mushroom with royal jelly, codonopsis, and lycium berries, and *Feng Ru Jiang*, royal jelly with codonopsis and astragalus. *Bei Jing Feng Wang Jiang* contains royal jelly only. All four are general tonics, but especially suited for deficient *chi*.

Common name: Schizandra berries
Botanical name: *Schizandra sinensis*
Chinese name: *wu wei zi*
Principal use: tonic astringent
Organs affected: Lung, Kidney
Temperature: warm
Contraindications: heat signs, pregnancy
Dose: 6–9 grams

Schizandra, which appeared in the oldest book of Chinese medicine, is most commonly used in Chinese medicine as an astringent for such symptoms as diarrhea or excessive sweating that often accompany deficiency syndromes. It has tonic properties of its own, reducing nervous exhaustion, building endurance, strengthening the reflexes, and increasing work efficiency. It also has sedative properties useful for insomnia due to deficiency. It is included in Chinese formulas for low energy, insomnia, diarrhea, sexual weakness, involuntary sweating, tuberculosis, asthma, and diabetes.

In a Chinese clinical trial, alcohol extracts of schizandra were given to 73 patients suffering from neurasthenia (nervous exhaustion). Forty-three patients were cured, and 13 significantly improved.

If taken alone and in high doses, schizandra can cause restlessness and insomnia. It also contains bitter substances called tannins. These are probably partly responsible for its astringent properties. For tonic use, I soak the berries for a few hours to reduce the bitterness, drain the water, and then dry them again. The soaked berries can be further allowed to soak in wine for several weeks, to make an excellent tonic for the Kidney.

Schizandra is available in bulk in Chinese stores, or through the mail. It is not usually used alone. Some possible combinations:

schizandra with codonopsis
schizandra with astragalus
schizandra with lycium berries and licorice
schizandra with rehmannia

Common name: Tienchi ginseng, Sanchi ginseng
Botanical name: *Panax pseudoginseng*
Chinese names: *tienchi, sanchi*
Primary uses: trauma medicine
Secondary use: *chi* tonic
Organs affected: Liver, Stomach, Large Intestine
Temperature: warm
Contraindications: pregnancy, caution in deficient blood
Dose: 1–3 grams of powder; 3–9 grams of root for tea

A preparation of this close relative of ginseng was standard issue to North Vietnamese troops during the Vietnam War. Although soldiers in Asia have, from time to time, used Chinese ginseng to increase endurance during combat, this herb was used for a very different purpose: it reduces bleeding. The soldiers used it as first aid for gunshot wounds until they could receive medical attention. It is also used in Chinese hospitals for serious bleeding in the gastrointestinal tract, the lungs, or from the nose.

I first became aware of tienchi when I tore some ligaments in my shoulder while playing basketball. Over the course of two days, an ugly bruise from internal bleeding spread from my shoulder all the way down to my elbow. My acupuncturist gave me some tienchi ginseng in a powdered form; the internal bleeding promptly stopped, the pain decreased, and the bruise resolved quickly. Tienchi is also used for sprains, strains, painful menstruation, and other kinds of external or internal bleeding when the blood is congealed into bruises.

Tienchi is used in China for heart-attack patients and others with coronary artery disease. Clinical trials there show that it increases the blood flow through the coronary arteries and lowers cholesterol levels.

Tienchi contains some of the same constituents as its close relative, ginseng, and is sometimes used as a general tonic as well. In a clinical trial, it was used along with chemotherapy for cancer, and improved the success of that treatment. Tienchi increases the efficiency of circulatory function in athletes. In trials with weight lifters and swimmers, it was found to lower maximum heart rates and hasten the return to a normal pulse after exercise. It might be a preferred tonic for athletes in contact sports, because it both increases efficiency and helps resolve bruises and swellings.

Tienchi is available in bulk, powdered, sliced, or in whole roots, from Spring Wind. Whole roots are also available from East Earth Tradewinds and from some Chinese stores. The prepared medicine I took for my torn shoulder is called *Yunnan Paiyao*. It comes as a powder in small vials, with a red pill on top of the bottle, or as capsules. The pill is only for cases of severe bleeding and traumatic shock, not for normal athletic trauma. For external bleeding, the powder can be sprinkled directly in a wound or taken in water. For strains, sprains, bruises, or gynecological bleeding, take it with some wine. *Yunnan Paiyao* is available in any Chinese

store, or through East Earth Tradewinds or the Institute
for Traditional Medicine. It is an excellent addition to a first
aid kit.

Adjuvant Herbs: Movers and Shakers

Several herbs that are not themselves tonics are often
found in tonic formulas. They are added in order to improve
the digestion and to promote circulation of the *chi* and blood
generated by the tonic herbs. Most are warming in nature,
and are circulatory stimulants. Remember that poor digestion often accompanies deficiency syndromes, and that one of
the major disorders of *chi* is stuck *chi* that does not flow properly. These adjuvant herbs help to solve both problems.
Licorice and/or jujube dates, which I've covered in their own
sections in this chapter, are added to many tonic formulas
both as adjuvant digestion-promoting herbs, and as minor
tonics in their own right. Some others are listed below:

Citrus peel (*chen pi*)   These are the dried peels of Chinese
species of oranges or tangerines. Citrus peel is both warming and bitter. It aids in digestion and promotes circulation of
chi. Citrus peel is readily available in Chinese stores, and
orange peel, its equivalent, is available in Western herb
stores.

Ginger root (*sheng chiang*)   Dried ginger root is a powerful
warming digestive herb. It has strong anti-nausea properties, and has been found in clinical trials to be as effective
for nausea as the conventional drug Dramamine, which
is often prescribed for motion sickness. Other trials
have shown that it can reduce or eliminate the nausea that

accompanies chemotherapy. Ginger may be included in tonic formulas when poor digestion and cold signs predominate. A classic *chi* and blood tonic formula from Chinese medicine uses both ginger and citrus peel:

he shou wu	2-3 parts	blood and yin tonic
ginseng	2 parts	*chi* tonic
(or codonopsis, 4 parts)		
dong quai	1 part	blood tonic
citrus peel	1 part	adjuvant
dried ginger	1 part	adjuvant

Ligusticum (*chuan xiong*)   Ligusticum is an acrid herb that promotes circulation of both blood and *chi*. It is often combined with blood tonics to promote circulation. It is a part of the Four Things Decoction, the most famous blood tonic formula in Chinese medicine (See *dong quai*) where it is included as an adjuvant to the three tonic herbs in the formula.

Bupleurum (*chai-hu*)   Bupleurum is considered a liver herb in Chinese medicine, but remember that the Chinese concept of Liver includes the regulation of the flow of blood, *chi*, and emotions. The syndrome of *stuck liver chi*, which is very common in Westerners, includes feelings of anger and frustration. Bupleurum, a cooling herb, is sometimes added to strong tonic formulas, such as those for athletes, in order to ensure that the generated *chi* moves harmoniously and to counteract metabolic heat generated by the tonic herbs.

Contraindications

Heat signs   The following herbs are contraindicated for use alone in a person with heat signs (See Table 4.2). They might be used with caution in formulas with other herbs that have a predominantly cooling effect.

> Asian ginseng
> deer antler
> astragalus
> atractylodes
> *dong quai*
> eleuthero root
> eucommia
> morindae
> schizandra
> citrus peel
> ginger
> ligusticum

Cold signs   The following herbs are contraindicated for use alone in a person with cold signs (See Table 4.2). They might be used with caution in formulas with other herbs that have a predominantly warming effect.

> asparagus
> dendrobium
> glehnia
> peony

Abdominal bloating   The following herbs are contraindicated for use alone in a person with abdominal bloating. They might be used with caution in formulas with other herbs that are Spleen tonics or digestive stimulants.

American ginseng
dendrobium
Fo Ti
jujube dates
lycium berries
rehmannia

For a table summarizing the actions of the tonic herbs see Appendix C.

How to Use Ginseng and the Tonic Herbs

If you think that you have one of the deficiency syndromes I described in the last section, or if you are under unusual stress, or if you are an athlete trying to build your performance and endurance, you may want to use ginseng and other tonic herbs. In this section, I will describe how to do so. But first, let me give an overview on treating deficiency conditions.

Americans usually take drugs with the expectation that the drug will make them better. Taking an aspirin for a headache, a blood-pressure medication for hypertension, or an antidepressant for depression might help your condition. This approach won't work with ginseng and other tonic herbs. Western drugs may address particular symptoms, but they don't act to build up the whole system. In fact, most of them weaken overall vitality while suppressing a symptom. The benefit of tonic herbs is that they can do for the overall system what no pharmaceutical drug can do.

The tonic herbs, unlike pharmaceutical drugs, are not fast-acting. They usually take two weeks to two months to produce their effects. But, more important, their use should be seen in a larger context. The solution to general deficiency is to change the patterns that are causing it, and no herb or formula can accomplish such a huge task by itself. Deficiency states are an overall problem, brought about by conditions in the diet, sleep patterns, stimulant use, stress-management habits, exercise habits, mental attitudes, and other lifestyle factors. As discussed in Section I, the Chinese use ginseng and other tonic herbs in the context of a lifestyle that cultivates and supports the *chi*. You'll have to do the same in order to achieve the results you want. Rather than view tonic herbs as drugs that will solve your problems, view them as allies that will help you to build a healthier lifestyle.

In this section, I'll describe some of the conditions for which ginseng might be helpful. Then I'll go into details about how to use ginseng and some tonic herbs, including dosage, duration, preparation, and time of year. I'll suggest some simple formulas you can make or purchase for yourself. Finally, I'll devote a chapter to how athletes might use ginseng and the tonic herbs.

CHAPTER 14

WHEN TO TAKE GINSENG AND THE TONIC HERBS

"Tonics should not be used indiscriminately like vitamins just because 'everyone can use a little tonification.' Side effects will often develop when tonics are prescribed for individuals who are not suffering from deficiency."

Dan Bensky, O.M.D., D.O.,
co-author of Chinese Herbal Medicine
Materia Medica

In this chapter, I'll give practical suggestions for taking ginseng. But first let's look at some precautions.

ARE YOU SICK?

If you have an illness, especially a chronic one, it is not wise to treat yourself with ginseng or other tonic herbs. Chronic illnesses are complex in both their causes and their presentation. The Chinese never treat such illnesses with ginseng alone, although they might include it in a formula tailored to

191

your specific condition. If you are sick, I suggest that you get a complete medical checkup. In the case I presented in Chapter 7, a man with chronic low energy and depression self-prescribed ginseng inappropriately when he was suffering from a vitamin deficiency. Ginseng isn't a vitamin, although it will boost your energy (and you might take vitamins along with it). You can easily mask the symptoms of a more serious underlying illness or nutrient deficiency with ginseng. The condition may then continue to get worse even though your energy level is better when taking ginseng.

If you want to avoid conventional medical treatment and use tonic herbs instead, you might consult an acupuncturist or other practitioner of Chinese medicine. I've provided referral numbers in Appendix B. Taking ginseng is never appropriate if you are experiencing an acute illness such as a cold or flu, or if you have allergies or aggravated arthritis. Please review the material in Chapter 7 on the contraindications for taking ginseng.

Are You "Stressed"?

Ginseng, eleuthero root, and other tonic herbs help the system to handle stressful situations. But stress means different things to different people. Fatigue, anxiety, insomnia, depression, tension, headache, and irritability all fall under the category of stress symptoms in the public view. From the point of view of Chinese medicine, however, these symptoms might fall into two groups. Tension, headaches, irritability, or depression may be due to a condition of excess, or to *chi* that is stuck and not flowing properly. Ginseng and other tonics will probably make the condition worse. Fatigue, anxiety, and insomnia, on the other hand, are common symptoms of deficiency, and ginseng or other tonic herbs might help. Depression could fall into either category. Use the Tables in Chapter 4 to asses your condition, rather than relying on your usual definition of stress.

DIGESTION

We saw in Chapters 2 and 5 how important good digestion is to maintaining the overall vitality of the *chi* and blood. It is a common practice in Chinese medicine to first address digestive problems before giving tonic herbs, or to include digestive stimulant herbs in tonic formulas. In my years of practice using Western herbs, I have often seen seriously ill patients regain their vitality by taking a simple digestive herb formula, without the need to take tonics at all. The standard American diet is very hard on the digestive system, and many Americans have become so accustomed to having indigestion that they think it is normal. Below are some common signs of a poorly functioning digestive system:

- flatulence or belching
- nausea
- pain anywhere in the digestive tract
- undigested food in the stool
- offensive breath
- constipation (less than one bowel movement per day)
- lethargy or depression after meals
- food cravings other than normal hunger
- lack of satisfaction after meals
- lack of hunger for breakfast

If you have any of these conditions, I suggest that you take the following formula of Western herbs for three to six weeks, and see if your overall health and energy improve. Take equal parts of chamomile, peppermint, fennel seed, licorice root, and burdock root. Put a handful of each in a pot and add two quarts of water. Simmer over low heat, with a lid on the pot, for one half hour. Strain and store for future use, in a thermos if you have one. Let this be your beverage, and drink at least three cups a day.

A handy way to make this, if you have a drip coffee maker, is to put the herbs in the pot (not the strainer) and add water in the back of the coffee maker. Turn it on. The hot water then flows onto the herbs, and the hot plate keeps the herbs at a good simmering temperature without boiling them. You can keep the tea hot on the coffee maker throughout the day, or strain it and put it into a thermos to take to work. You can also add fresh water to the used herbs once, as there will still be plenty of potency left in the once-brewed herbs. It's important to make enough of this tea in advance, so that you don't have to hassle with brewing the tea each time you want a cup. Otherwise, you probably won't keep up the practice long enough to obtain the benefits you want.

Deficiency, Absolute and Relative

The Chinese say not to take ginseng unless you are deficient. I covered deficiency states in detail in Chapter 4. This approach is changing in Korea and Japan however, where people in normal health take daily ginseng doses to combat the unremitting stress of modern society. You might say that, like athletes, many of us are healthy but are deficient relative to the demands put on us by jobs, families, and the environment. I think if you are normally healthy, you can take minimum doses of ginseng, provided that you do not show signs of excess or heat (see Chapter 4) and as long as you know how to watch for the signs of adverse effects that might appear (Chapter 7). If you do develop adverse effects, stop completely for a few weeks, then try again at half the dose.

Below are some circumstances under which you might find ginseng or eleuthero root helpful. Ginseng is superior to eleuthero root as an overall tonic, but eleuthero is much less expensive and has been shown in scientific research to be effective for the conditions listed. Start taking it at least three weeks in advance if possible.

- When you foresee a very stressful period, such as a job change, moving to a new city or climate, or increased family responsibilities.
- When the seasons change. Physicians know that colds and flu tend to occur most often when the weather changes. If the weather is suddenly turning cold or windy, consider taking astragalus along with the ginseng. Or make a tonic soup (I provided a recipe in Chapter 13 under "codonopsis"). Tonic soup mixes are a regular commodity in Chinese stores, and the Chinese frequently use them when the seasons change.
- During periods when you are prone to catch cold. Note that eleuthero root is widely used to prevent colds in Russia.
- When traveling or moving to a higher altitude. Ginseng or eleuthero can increase aerobic capacity. Ginseng is superior to eleuthero for this purpose, because it also helps build the blood.

- When driving on a long journey. Instead of pumping coffee to stay alert, start taking ginseng in advance. If you haven't started before the trip, ginseng in doses of over three grams has an effect similar to that of caffeine, but does not deplete the system.
- To combat jet lag.
- If you are under a temporarily demanding work schedule, such as a deadline for a project.
- If you will have to stay up all night for some reason. Take the ginseng before your all-nighter, and for a few days afterward to help you recover.
- When you're temporarily tired and worn out. If this is a chronic condition, have a medical checkup.
- If you are over 40 and begin to feel the effects of aging.

DOSAGE AND DURATION

Use a minimum dose of ginseng and other herbs for a long time rather than a high dose for a short time. I provided dose ranges for each of the herbs in Chapter 13. The upper ranges are for use by practitioners with training in Chinese medicine. Wait three weeks before deciding whether the ginseng is helping you. You might make a list of your physical and psychological symptoms when you start. Then make another list after three weeks and compare them. Other tonic formulas may show effects in three days to a week, but give them about two weeks to do their work. Some will cause minor side effects in the first few days that will disappear soon. Continue taking the formula for up to a month if you do not develop long-term side effects. Some single herbs, including cordyceps, Prince ginseng, eleuthero root, tienchi ginseng,

Fo-Ti, asparagus, and dendrobium might be taken long-term, provided that they do not evoke adverse effects.

Even if you don't experience side effects, take a break from the ginseng for a week or two every few months. Also, take breaks during very hot weather, because ginseng can heat up the system. The Chinese most often take ginseng as a regular tonic during the colder winter months, and during season changes as fall turns to winter and winter turns to spring. In very hot summer weather, consider taking American ginseng, which is cooling and also helps relieve fatigue. For other tonic herb formulas, take a week-long break every four to six weeks.

TIPS

Some other tips for taking ginseng and tonic herbs:

- Take them on an empty stomach.
- Prepare a formula that includes digestive aids. Combine licorice, jujube dates, citrus peel, or ginger with ginseng or other herbs.
- Use ginseng and other tonics to restore normal function rather than to drive your system to unnatural heights.

In Chapter 15, I'll tell you ways to prepare ginseng and tonic herb formulas.

How to Prepare Ginseng and Tonic Herbs

You can take ginseng and other herbs in six main forms: raw, slightly cooked, or as a tea, wine, powder, or extract.

Ginseng Roots

Whole ginseng roots are readily available in Chinese stores or through the mail. I'll list mail-order sources in Appendix A. One advantage to buying ginseng roots whole is that at least you know you have ginseng. We'll see in Chapter 17 that many products in stores either contain no ginseng at all, or contain amounts too small to do you any good. Ginseng comes in many grades, and some are much more potent than others. If you are buying from a reputable dealer, the medicinal quality will be reflected by the price. Better ginseng costs more, and sometimes a lot more. "Let the buyer beware" is the rule if you buy ginseng roots in stores, however. Western store owners often do not know how to buy good quality roots, and some Chinese dealers will try to pass off an inexpensive root to the naive buyer as a higher quality one. I'll describe the grades of roots in Chapter 18, and provide you with information on reputable dealers in Appendix A.

Eating Ginseng

Eating ginseng raw or lightly steamed has the advantage that you know you are getting all the constituents. Whole roots are hard to cut; if you steam them for a few minutes, cutting is easier. Cut them in slices about the thickness of a nickel. Cut up the whole root, or it will dry out and you'll have to steam it again. The dose for the average person is one or two of these thin slices a day. I pour honey over the sliced roots and keep them in the refrigerator in a closed container, then take them as I need them. You can also buy the root in a pre-sliced form. Some Korean products come in this form; you can also purchase root slices from Spring Wind. The slices are gram for gram less expensive than the whole root.

Don't even think about eating a whole large root! We saw in Chapter 6 that one-ounce (30-gram) doses of ginseng are used in hospitals to revive patients in life-threatening shock, or to temporarily revive the terminally ill. Such a dose would surely be overstimulating to a healthy person. The weights of individual roots that I have seen range from about five grams to an ounce. My buying experience is limited, however, and you should weigh whatever roots you have; aim for a one-to-two-gram dose. If you don't have a gram scale, use a postage or diet scale that measures ounces. See how many roots it takes to reach 1 ounce. There are about 30 grams in an ounce, so divide 30 by the number of roots it takes to reach an ounce to find the number of grams in each root. If it takes 5 roots to reach 1 ounce, for example, they weigh about 6 grams each. Some whole roots weigh an entire ounce.

POWDERED GINSENG

The way I prefer to eat ginseng is to grind up a root in a coffee or seed grinder to make a powder. I can then add a gram or two of the powder to some warm water or a small glass of wine, stir it well, and drink. Ginseng is easier to digest in this form than are the root slices. You can also put the powder in gelatin capsules, which are available in most health food stores. They are available from East Earth Tradewinds or Frontier Herbs. Both companies sell capsule fillers which allow you to fill 50 or more capsules at once. You can also mix the ginseng powder with other powdered herbs to make a formula. Ginseng powders can be purchased in stores or through the mail, but I recommend that you powder your own to ensure the highest quality.

TEAS

Making a tea of the roots has the advantage that you can easily mix other herbs with it. It is common in China to add three to five jujube dates to a ginseng root tea. Other herbs, such as licorice root, astragalus, *Fo-Ti*, *dong quai*, or schizandra berries, can also be added to make a simple tonic formula.

Ginseng is much too expensive to prepare like a regular tea. It should be cooked in a covered double boiler. The Chinese use a small porcelain container called a ginseng cooker, which takes the place of the top portion of a double boiler. It holds enough water for about two cups of tea. It has an inner lid that covers the top to keep valuable ginseng constituents from evaporating, and a second domed lid that fits over that, creating an insulating air space between the first and the second lids. These cookers are quite inexpensive and can be found in any Chinese store, or they can be ordered through the mail from East Earth Tradewinds. You can also use a pint canning jar with a lid for the same purpose by placing the covered jar with its ginseng and water contents in a large pot of boiling water. The point of the cooker or jar is to keep the ginseng tea from boiling, which can cause the loss of some of its constituents.

Use about six grams of ginseng and some water in the cooker or in a jar in a pot of boiling water, and cook the tea for about two hours, adding water to the pot as it boils away if necessary. If you don't want to worry about watching the water level, use a crock pot on a low setting instead of a pot on the stove. Cook the ginseng about an hour longer in the crock pot than you would on the stove.

Remove the tea, and drink half of it as a daily dose. Don't throw away the ginseng root and other herbs yet. The first boiling extracts the constituents from the outer part of the root, but does not reach the interior. To prepare for the second boiling, cut the root up into small slices, exposing the core of the root. Then repeat the cooking process two more times, for a total of three boilings. Thus you can get six doses of the tea from a single root. If you start to feel overstimulated by this dose, or start to develop any of the adverse effects of ginseng, take a break for a week, and repeat taking a fourth or a third of the contents of the cooker or jar as a daily dose.

Other Tonic Teas

The above method is best for ginseng because it is such an expensive herb. For other tonic herbs, it is customary to simmer them directly in a pot rather than using a double boiler. The softer herbs and leafy herbs require only 20 to 30 minutes. For roots and harder substances, and for formulas, simmer them on a low flame until about a third or half the water has evaporated. They are then ready for use. As with ginseng, you can repeat the process three times, breaking up any hard root for the second boiling. If your formula includes ginseng and many other herbs, prepare the ginseng in a double boiler, and the other herbs in this manner, then mix the two liquids.

Ginseng Wines

In China, a common way to take ginseng and some other tonic herbs is to soak them in wine and then drink the wine. The traditional liquor is rice wine, but any wine or strong liquor will do. Wine itself is considered medicinal in China, in doses of an ounce. Wines "moves" the blood, promoting circulation, and thus makes a good complement to tonic herbs.

To make a ginseng-wine preparation, chop or thinly slice about three ounces of ginseng root and let them soak in the liquor for five or six weeks. Keep the mixture in a dark, cool place, and shake it up every day or two. When it's ready, remember that this is a medicine, and not a regular alcoholic beverage. Overindulgence can easily cause overstimulation.

Other tonic herbs that are suitable for making such wines are deer antler, eleuthero root, *Fo-Ti*, schizandra berries, and rehmannia. Add a little fennel seed or cardamom along with rehmannia to promote digestion and circulation. You can also mix these herbs with ginseng in the wine.

PREPARED PRODUCTS

Ginseng is available in a wide variety of forms in stores: powders, capsules, granules, teas, liquid extracts, and more. The products vary widely in potency, ranging from worthless to very strong. It is often hard to tell from the label exactly what strength of ginseng is inside. Ginseng products that come from Korea, widely available in health food stores, tend to be of good quality. I mentioned some excellent American products under Ginseng in Chapter 13. For all prepared products, follow the instructions on the label.

OTHER TONIC FORMULAS

I described how to prepare tonic formulas in the above paragraphs under Powders, Teas, and Wines. Hundreds of tonic formulas are now available in the American marketplace. I've described some of them in Chapter 13. Refer to Appendix A for a list of companies that make high-quality tonic formulas.

CHAPTER 16

ATHLETES
AND THE
TONIC HERBS

I was a distance runner and soccer player when I was younger, and experienced the ups and downs of training, racing, and injuries for many years. On several occasions, I overtrained and experienced "runner's burnout." On one occasion, I collapsed with heat exhaustion after racing a hilly course on an unseasonably hot spring day. I experienced many sprains, a few breaks, and some severely torn ligaments. I was forced to stop competing at around age 40 because of soccer injuries. I wish that I had known, during my nearly 30 years of athletic competition, what I now know about ginseng and the tonic herbs. They could have enhanced my performance, aided regeneration after competition, and helped me recover from injuries.

In general, tonic herbs should only be used for people in a state of deficiency, but serious athletes have their own special brand of deficiency states. They are generally deficient relative to their level of activity. They create states of deficiency and exhaustion through heavy training and all-out competition. My normal state upon crossing the finish line in 10-kilometer races was to be short of breath, weak in the legs, sweating profusely, feeling faint, and completely exhausted, with spots before my eyes and a foggy mind — symptoms of deficiency in *chi*, yin, yang and blood! I know now that ginseng and tonic herbs can help to increase one's performance level before that state is reached, and can hasten recovery after a competition. The tonics can build energy, endurance, blood, muscle, and aerobic capacity. They help me now as I limp about the racquetball court! Here are a few suggestions for athletes.

Ginseng and Aerobic Capacity

Athletic activity depends greatly on the aerobic capacity of the athlete: the ability to utilize oxygen efficiently. This depends on respiratory activity, but also on the chemical state of the tissues that utilize the oxygen, and on physiological changes such as increasing the capacity of the heart muscle and the action and efficiency of tiny blood vessels that circulate oxygenated blood to the cells. Trials in both humans and animals have shown that Chinese ginseng greatly increases aerobic capacity. Other tonic herbs, including tienchi ginseng and eleuthero root, have similar action.

Animal research on ginseng, tienchi, and eleuthero root showed that animals treated with the herbs and then subjected to very low atmospheric pressure (low oxygen content) survive longer than animals not treated. Likewise, a group of Chinese workers transferred to an elevation of

14,000 feet in Tibet suffered less from oxygen-deficit after taking these herbs than did untreated workers. Animals subjected to vigorous exercise can perform up to 100% longer when treated with ginseng. They also utilize less of their stored glycogen, the ready source of energy stored in the liver. Marathon runners who "hit the wall" and run out of energy toward the end of their race do so because they have exhausted their glycogen supplies. Glycogen-loading—eating high-carbohydrate meals before a competition to build up glycogen—is a common practice among endurance athletes. Ginseng could increase performance by reducing the requirements for glycogen.

All three herbs have also been tested on athletes, and have been shown to increase aerobic capacity. In a Swiss trial with Asian ginseng, athletes were first tested for maximum heart rate and recovery time in an eight-minute exercise test. Their average heart rate increased from 70 beats per minute to more than 150 beats. Their heart rates fell below 100 beats per minute within five minutes, and returned to normal in about twenty minutes. They then took ginseng for nine weeks. After that time, the same exercise increased the heart rate to only 140 beats per minute. More dramatically, the rates then fell below 100 beats within three minutes instead of the usual five, and returned to normal within five minutes instead of the original twenty.

The lactate levels of the athletes were tested during the same trials. Lactate is a by-product of aerobic activity that causes muscle pain after exercise. After ginseng treatment, peak lactate levels fell by 40%, and returned to normal faster than before treatment.

Different levels of ginseng were tested in these athletes, and no advantage was found to taking unusually high doses of ginseng. The beneficial effects of the ginseng persisted for up to three weeks after the nine-week course. Another Swiss study showed that benefits to aerobic capacity, although present in all age groups tested, are most pronounced in the 40–60 age group, supporting the traditional Chinese wisdom that ginseng is especially beneficial for those over 40.

In China, similar benefits were found in weight lifters and swimmers who took tienchi ginseng. After a day of heavy training, weight lifters' pulse rates often do not return to normal even by the next morning, but they will do so after taking tienchi. Swimmers' maximum heart rates after training were reduced from 170 beats per minute to 125. Their recovery time was also dramatically reduced. Without tienchi, their pulse rates fell to about 120 beats per minute after 2 to 3 minutes.

After taking tienchi for seven weeks, their pulses returned to their normal resting rates, about 70 beats, in the same time. When compared to swimmers not taking the tienchi, these differences in aerobic capacity increased steadily throughout the seven weeks.

Dosage

If you want to take ginseng alone, use low doses for long periods rather than high doses for short periods when preparing for competition. The medicinal dose of ginseng is one to nine grams; I suggest that athletes take one or two grams for several months at a time. The reason is that athletes, although they experience states of deficiency during training and competition, are generally close to the edge of being in excess. Normal medicinal doses of ginseng can throw such a system over the line and produce symptoms such as muscle tension, insomnia, headaches, and heat signs—not what the athlete is looking for. The lower doses are less likely to do this, but will gradually build the endurance and reflexes.

Eleuthero root and tienchi ginseng are both valuable tonics for athletes, and are less likely to produce symptoms of excess than is Chinese ginseng. A low-range dose for eleuthero is five grams (about a sixth of an ounce). Eleuthero is readily available in bulk in health food stores or from the bulk herb suppliers listed in Appendix A. The dose for eleuthero tincture (a quarter- to a half-ounce a day) can be prohibitively expensive. More concentrated, and thus more affordable, eleuthero extracts are available from Gaia herbs, HerbPharm, or McZand Herbals.

Tienchi ginseng is harder to find, but is available in bulk from East Earth Tradewinds or Spring Wind. Russian athletes sometimes combine all three herbs.

American ginseng is also a valuable tonic for summer sports, because it cools excess heat while helping to reduce fatigue. It is even more expensive than Chinese ginseng. The best bulk prices are from White Crane and Spring Wind. The dose is three grams. Excellent concentrated extracts are produced by Gaia Herbs and HerbPharm.

USE GINSENG IN A FORMULA

In China, athletes do not take ginseng alone, but rather in formulas that combine *chi*, blood, and other tonics. Chinese women distance runners in the last Olympic games performed so well—breaking every record in women's long distance running—that they were suspected of using steroids or other drugs to boost their performance. Their coach denied this, and their urine tests for drugs came out negative. The coach said that all they took was some traditional tonic herbal formulas.

The following formula was devised by an American company for athletes competing in the 1984 Olympic Trials and Summer Olympics in Los Angeles, California. Under the name Active Herbal, it is available from McZand Herbals.

Eleuthero (Siberian ginseng)
American ginseng
Astragalus
Ginkgo
Fo-Ti
Licorice

The eleuthero root increases aerobic capacity, endurance, and reaction time. American ginseng was probably included because it was summertime. American ginseng reduces heat, and also strengthens the lungs. Astragalus strengthens the lungs and builds both *chi* and blood. Ginkgo leaf is not a traditional Chinese herb, but it increases peripheral circulation, including circulation to the brain. *Fo-Ti* is a powerful blood tonic, and strengthens the Kidney (aiding in endurance) and the Liver (helping the smooth circulation of *chi* and blood). Licorice strengthens the Spleen, which is responsible for muscle strength, and also helps circulate the benefits of the formula into all the meridians.

If you are a serious athlete, I suggest that you consult an acupuncturist or other Chinese practitioner for a personalized formula. It is a small investment to get a tonic formula tailored to your own physique, your training level, and the needs of your particular sport. Champion Chinese and

Russian athletes don't take single herbs or off-the-shelf formulas to enhance their performance. I suggest getting one formula to prepare for competition, one for around the time or on the day of the competition itself, and then another for recovery.

THE SPLEEN AND ATHLETICS

We saw in Chapter 5 that the Chinese Spleen organ is responsible for transforming food into *chi*, then sending this to the Lung, where it is mixed with *chi* from the air to produce blood. The Spleen also nourishes the muscles, and Spleen tonics are very important for building athletic performance. Ginseng is a Spleen tonic, and this is responsible for some of its benefits for athletes. The following formula, devised by herbalist Ron Teeguarden and available from East Earth Tradewinds, focuses on tonification of the Spleen and building overall energy and muscle strength.

Athlete's Tonic

Chinese ginseng	3 parts	*chi* and Spleen tonic
Astragalus	3 parts	*chi* and Lung tonic
Atractylodes	3 parts	Spleen tonic
Bupleurum	2 parts	prevents stagnation of *chi*
Citrus peel	2 parts	Spleen tonic, promotes circulation of *chi*
Ginger	2 parts	Spleen tonic
Jujube dates	2 parts	Spleen tonic, *chi* tonic
Licorice	2 parts	benefits lungs and digestion, promotes flow of *chi* in all the meridians

Training

Of the three phases in the cycle of athletics—training, competition, and recovery—training takes the most time. It is also the most important, because performance during competition depends mainly on training. Reflexes and mental attitude may be more important during competition, but success depends on repeatedly conditioning the reflexes and building a strong circulatory system, muscle mass, and connective tissue during training. Thus, this is the most important time to be taking ginseng and other tonic herbs.

Of great concern to athletes, whether in contact or endurance sports, is building up muscle mass. A marathon runner beginning training spends months running long distances at slow speeds and doing hill-work in order to build muscle volume. Muscle volume is equally important for the weight lifter, football player, distance runner, or sprinter. This is why athletes take anabolic steroids, which build muscle mass and increase aggressive energy. Of course, these drugs are banned in formal competition. They linger in the system for a long time, and may be evident in urine tests even months after stopping their use. Chinese tonic herbs can also help build muscle mass, but they do so more harmoniously, do not present the health risks of steroids, and are legal in competition. A practitioner of Chinese medicine would say that steroids deplete the internal organs by transferring their *chi* to the muscles. Chinese tonics strengthen the internal organs themselves, and benefit the muscles indirectly. The Chinese women distance runners I mentioned above raised eyebrows at the Olympics because of their well-developed musculature and their high tolerance for unusually rigorous training exercises.

To understand how tonic herbs can do this, let's look again at the Chinese Kidney. Part of the Kidney function corresponds to that of the adrenal glands. These glands are important for endurance, and they also release the stress hormones — natural steroids that occur within the body. The Kidney is also important for growth. Kidney tonics are given to children who fail to grow properly. They can also help an athlete "grow" muscles. Kidney tonics also strengthen the bones and connective tissue, the lower back, and the knees. They raise the general metabolic rate, and increase the metabolism of sugars. Finally, the Kidney assists the lungs in breathing, and strong healthy Kidney function is necessary for good "wind."

The following formula from Jade Chinese Herbals, called Antler/Athletic, is the Rolls Royce of athletic training formulas. Jade has a series of formulas specifically for athletes, and I recommend that you get their catalogue. I will give details on how to contact them in Appendix A. The majority of herbs included in this formula are warming yang tonics that benefit both the Kidney and the Liver. The Liver controls the smooth flow of *chi* and blood, and ensures that energy and nutrition derived from the formula circulates harmoniously.

Antler/Athletic Training Formula:

Asian ginseng

Increases *chi*, tonifies the Spleen (which governs muscle strength) and Lung, builds the blood, and enhances endurance, aerobic capacity, conditioned learning, and mental clarity.

Epididimii

Tonifies the Kidney in a balanced way, and also benefits the Liver.

Eucommia

Strengthens Kidney and Liver function.

Drynaria

Tonifies the Kidney and the Heart, invigorates blood
circulation, strengthens the tendons, and suppresses pain.

Morindae

Tonifies the Kidney. Strengthens muscles and bones.

Polygonum(*Fo-Ti*)

Strengthens the Kidney and Liver, builds the blood.

Poria

Strengthens the Spleen, thus enhancing muscle
strength.

Deer antler

Tonifies both *chi* and blood. Strengthens Kidney and
Liver. Contains natural testosterone-like sterols. Strengthens
bones and promotes growth.

Antelope horn

Strong cooling properties balance the other warming
herbs in the formula. Antelope horn also increases aerobic
capacity.

The formula contains tonics for *chi* and blood, herbs
to develop both the yang and the yin of the Kidney, herbs
for the Liver to promote the smooth flow of blood and *chi*,
and Spleen tonics to increase the strength of the muscles.

A similar but much simpler formula, created by herbalist Ron Teeguarden and available from East Earth Tradewinds, is Vital Essence Formula. It contains high-quality
ginseng, deer antler, schizandra berries, and lycium berries.

PERFORMANCE

Performance depends mainly on proper training, reflexes, mental clarity, and attitude. Ginseng, tienchi, and eleuthero root all improve the reflexes and mental clarity, but won't do much good if you start taking them the day before the event. Two to three months of treatment with them will increase these qualities to a high level. Two formulas from Jade Chinese Herbals are specifically designed for such quick effects and make a good supplement to long-term tonification. Black Belt is a combination of 35 herbs, and comes in a form like fruit leather. The other formula, called Energy, contains blood, *chi*, yin, and yang tonics with ephedra. Ephedra is a powerful stimulant, not appropriate for regular or long-term use. It can be very drying and overstimulating, and is banned in some athletic contests. This formula is devised to counterbalance the negative effects of ephedra.

RECOVERY

It is a general rule in distance running that, after a race, an athlete should rest by training lightly at less than the race pace for one day for every mile that was raced. Thus, runners wait about a week before training hard after a 10-kilometer race (6.6 miles), and about a month after a marathon (about 28 miles). Comparable recovery periods are necessary for most competitive sports that require exercise to exhaustion. You can easily hasten this recovery period using tonic herbs. One herb that can be used alone for this is cordyceps, which I covered in detail in Chapter 13. It is a Kidney tonic that is balanced in its energy—neither warming nor cooling—and can be taken for long periods. A recovery formula should include a balance of *chi*, yang, blood, and yin tonics. Another formula from Jade, Endurance, is well balanced. It has some herbs in common with the Antler/Athletic formula described above, but has blood and yin tonics added, and contains fewer yang tonics.

Endurance Formula:

Chinese ginseng	*chi* and yin tonic; builds blood, strengthens Spleen and Lung
Astragalus	*chi*, blood, and Lung tonic
Atractylodes	Spleen tonic
Deer antler	*chi*, blood, and yang tonic; strengthens Kidney and Liver
Dong quai	blood tonic; moves blood, moistens the organs
Eucommia	yang tonic for Kidney and Liver
Licorice	benefits lungs and digestion, promotes flow of *chi* in all the meridians
Lycium berries	blood and yin tonic for Liver and Kidney
Polygonum (*Fo-Ti*)	blood tonic for Liver and Kidney
Salvia	yin tonic for Heart and Kidney; moves blood
Schizandra	tonic for Kidney and Lung

This formula could be used for training as well. I mention it here because of its balance and its superiority over the other formulas mentioned for recovery from an exhausting competition. It should be taken for several weeks.

CONTACT SPORTS

The Swiss studies mentioned above show that ginseng, when taken for several months, improves reaction time. Other studies show that it aids conditioned learning. This can be especially effective for individuals in contact sports and the martial arts. Tienchi ginseng may be particularly appropriate for such events, because it aids in healing trauma, including sprains and bruises. See the discussion in Chapter 13 for more detail. The formulas under the subhead Performance above may also be useful on the day of the event.

SEASON, CLIMATE, AND ALTITUDE

Season is important to consider when taking ginseng and some other tonic herbs. In China, it is not unusual for people who take ginseng regularly to stop taking it during hot summer weather. This may be important for some athletes to consider as well because of ginseng's heating properties. It might be better to switch to tienchi or eleuthero as general tonics during summer. American ginseng is mostly untested for its ability to increase endurance, but in Chinese medicine it is not considered a significant *chi* tonic. It will reduce heat very well, which is why it is used to treat feverish diseases. Thus, American ginseng can be a good addition for training or performing when overheating might be a problem. This may apply as well when traveling to perform in a hot climate.

High altitude is another condition that can be the downfall of an athlete. Athletes who train at higher altitudes have greater aerobic capacity than those who train lower down. Within the U.S., teams training in Denver, which is more than a mile high, may have an advantage when playing at home over teams that train at sea level. Training at high altitude has been a great benefit to some African distance runners, who descend to lower altitudes to compete in world events. When moving or traveling to higher altitudes, an individual instantly develops the equivalent of a blood deficiency. This is responsible for the dizziness and the need for afternoon naps that is so common to new arrivals. After three to six weeks at a high altitude, an individual's red blood cell count will increase about 20% in order to handle the thinner air. Chinese ginseng, tienchi, and eleuthero root will all build aerobic capacity, and beginning to take them a month or two before an anticipated event at high altitude will improve performance. Combining the three, and taking them in double doses in the ten days before arrival, may also be helpful. Any formula that also includes blood tonics, such as Endurance above, may be of even greater benefit.

You don't need to be a world class athlete to use tonic herbs to enhance your performance and enjoyment of exercise. Even if you don't exercise vigorously, you might try any of the formulas or approaches to improve your experience of moderate exercise.

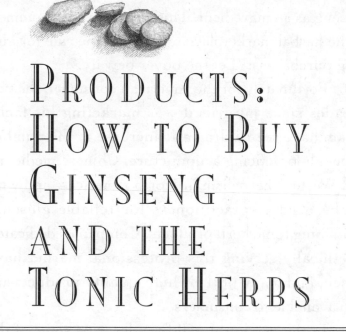

PRODUCTS: HOW TO BUY GINSENG AND THE TONIC HERBS

I have a friend who developed beauty products in the 1970s. One day, I saw that he was creating a "ginseng and aloe" facial cream. I asked him why he would put ginseng in a facial product, where it could not possibly have any beneficial effect. "Well," he responded with a shrug, "people are buying ginseng these days." As it turned out, he was putting in only a minute amount—just enough to "honestly" list ginseng as an ingredient. This attitude is still common in the herbal marketplace today, and the rule for ginseng purchase is: "Let the buyer beware."

Fortunately for the American consumer, the two decades since my friend was marketing his facial cream have seen a dramatic increase in the number of people practicing acupuncture, Chinese medicine, and Western herbalism in North America—and with it, the need of practitioners for reliable ginseng-containing tonic herb products. Companies dedicated to ethically serving this professional market have arisen, and many of their high-quality products are also available to consumers.

In this section, I will first describe some of the questionable areas, misleading marketing, and outright fraud surrounding the sale of ginseng in the U.S. today. I'll tell you how to buy whole ginseng roots intelligently, and I'll describe the kinds of products that are available.

CHAPTER 17

GINSENG SCAMS

In the late 1970s, several studies of ginseng products in the U.S. set off a bombshell in the health food industry. More than 50 of the most common ginseng products were analyzed for their contents; about 25% of them contained no ginseng at all, and another 35% contained so little ginseng as to be clinically worthless.

The situation has probably improved since the 1970s, but problems of fraud still remain. The November, 1995 *Consumer Reports* analyzed 10 ginseng products for their ginsenoside content. We saw in Chapter 9 that these substances are important active constituents in ginseng. Their presence in a product indicates that ginseng is present also, although higher levels do not necessarily indicate a better product because other constituents also contribute to ginseng's activity. A normal range of ginsenosides in a ginseng root is 3% to 6% by weight.

Table 17.1 ranks the products in the *Consumer Reports* study by percent of ginsenosides. I added the percentages

TABLE 17.1
ANALYSIS OF TEN COMMERCIAL GINSENG PRODUCTS*

Brand	Weight of the Tablet	Ginsenosides	% Ginsenosides
Walgreen's Gin-zing	100 mg	7.6 mg	7.60 %
Herbal Choice	100	6.5	6.50
American Ginseng	250	12.8	5.12
Ginsana	100	3.0	3.0
KRG	518	11.5	2.2
Solgar	520	10.6	2.00
Nature's Resource	560	10.7	1.91
GNC Natural Brand	648	3.6	0.56
Naturally	648	2.3	0.40
Rite Aid	250	0.4	0.02

*(Based on article in *Consumer Reports*, November, 1995)

myself; they did not appear in the original article. Six of the products apparently have less than 3% ginsenosides. Thus, their stated weight probably includes fillers and binders. Because some of these contain so little ginseng, they can have no medicinal effect. The other products contain ginseng, but their dosages can be confusing. Compare the weights in Table 17.1. The weight of the product from KRG appears to contain five times more ginseng than the products from Walgreen's or Herbal Choice. However, it is evident in the percentages of ginsenosides that these apparently stronger products instead contain fillers and binders and are not as potent.

DOSAGE SLEIGHT-OF-HAND

If we look at the products in another way, it is easier to rank them. The average minimum daily dose of ginsenosides should be about 30 to 60 milligrams a day, or an average of 45 milligrams, to get the equivalent of a one-gram tonic dose of ginseng. Table 17.2 shows the number of tablets of each of the products listed in Table 17.1 that you would have to take to get this dose. The American Ginseng brand, which appears to have only half the amount of ginseng of the next three brands on the list, actually delivers more ginsenosides.

Scientists working with the American Botanical Council (ABC) in Austin, Texas, are currently examining more than 100 ginseng products on the market for ginsenoside content. The results are expected to be ready for publication in late 1996. See the Resources section in the Appendix for how to contact the ABC if you would like to see the results. The ABC also publishes the *HerbalGram* magazine, and has the best available selection of mail-order books on herbs.

TABLE 17.2
ONE-GRAM GINSENG DOSES IN TABLETS

	Milligrams of Ginsenosides Per Tablet or Capsule	Tablets or Capsules to Get Equivalent of a One-Gram Dose of Ginseng
American Ginseng	12.8	4
KRG	11.5	5
Solgar	10.6	5
Nature's Resource	10.7	5
Walgreen's Gin-zing	7.6	7
Herbal Choice	6.5	8
GNC Natural Brand	3.6	14
Ginsana	3.0	17
Naturally	2.3	22
Rite Aid	0.4	125

GINSENOSIDE QUESTIONS

Many products available today are labeled "standardized for ginsenosides." Ginsenosides are like the fingerprints of ginseng; they prove that ginseng was at the scene of manufacture, but they don't tell how much ginseng was there, or, more important, what grade of ginseng was used to make the product. We saw in Chapter 9 that ginsenosides are not the only active constituents in ginseng, and that they are most concentrated in the root hairs, skin, and leaves of the ginseng plant. In Asia, where experts know the medicinal use of ginseng very well, these parts are trimmed off the plants and sold as inferior medicines. Asian scientific experts, fully aware of the research into ginsenosides, reject ginsenoside content as a predictor of medicinal activity. Instead, they choose ginseng by its grade and by the qualities I described in Chapter 9.

Two different grades of ginseng—for example, cultivated and semi-wild—may have identical ginsenoside content, but the semi-wild ginseng will be much more potent. If you ingest some of each root, the difference is evident very soon. Most companies that produce ginseng products for sale to the general public use the least expensive, lowest grade of ginseng they can find. These standardized products contain ginseng, but, as we saw above, most contain only a low dose. I'll explain ginseng grades in greater detail in Chapter 18.

Here is a summary of the misleading practices in ginseng-based American consumer products:

- Only trace amounts of ginseng in the product
- Too little ginseng to provide any medicinal benefit

- Weights of tablets manipulated to make them appear to contain more ginseng than they do
- Misleading labeling of ginsenoside content

The best way to tell if good-quality ginseng was used is by the price. Ginseng is the last product you want to bargain-hunt for. There are no ginseng bargains; better products will cost more.

GINSENG ROOT SCAMS

You can also run into major or minor fraud when buying roots in a shop. The most common scam is "the upgrade": selling a low-grade root as if it were a more expensive grade. If you don't know how to identify different grades of ginseng, it is impossible to avoid this unless you know the reputation of your supplier.

A famous scam in the ginseng trade is to take a wild American ginseng root, which looks much like wild Chinese ginseng, trim the root hairs from an inexpensive Chinese root, and weave or paste them onto the American root. It then looks like a very expensive Chinese root. True wild Chinese ginseng is extremely rare, and costs about $15,000 an ounce—that's $240,000 a pound! The fraudulent product also resembles semi-wild roots. These are not as valuable, but they are still so expensive that they are sold by the gram instead of the ounce.

ELEUTHERO ROOT ("SIBERIAN GINSENG")

Siberian ginseng may be subject to more fraud than even Asian ginseng. We saw in Chapter 13 that some confusion exists about identification of eleuthero root because several different species of plants in Asia traditionally have had the same Chinese name. One of them, *Periplocum sepium*, can produce toxic reactions. Some lots of "Siberian Ginseng" that have reached the U.S. have been found to be *periplocum* instead. Varro Tyler, Ph.D., reports in his book, *The Honest Herbal*, that the problem of misidentified eleuthero root is rampant. In one analysis of three lots of so-called eleuthero root, only one was found to contain any eleuthero at all, and that one was spiked with 5% caffeine! This problem exists at the level of the herb importer, and even well-intentioned companies may unwittingly buy and produce misidentified products.

Low dosing is another problem with eleuthero root tinctures. The Russian preparation that was used in the extensive research project mentioned in Chapter 13 was a tincture taken in doses ranging from 2 to 20 milliliters a day. That's between a sixteenth of an ounce and two-thirds of an ounce per day. Most tinctures come in one-ounce bottles priced at $7 to $10 each. The cost of taking such products in an effective dose over the long term would be prohibitive.

Furthermore, the Russian product is made with one part of eleuthero root in a solution of 30% alcohol (60% water). Most American tinctures are made with one part of eleuthero root to between two and five parts of 60% or more alcohol. They are thus much weaker than the Russian product. You would have to take two or three times more than the minimum two-milliliter dose to approximate the Russian dose.

Some American companies make very strong extracts of eleuthero that overcome this problem. Look on the label for a one-to-one or greater ratio of plant to solvent. The

HerbPharm company makes a product according to the Russian specifications, and then concentrates it so it is effectively twice as strong. With this product, you can use half the recommended dose to get the same results as the Russian researchers obtained. HerbPharm also makes an alcohol-free extract by first preparing the formula as usual, then evaporating the alcohol and adding glycerine and water.

COSMETICS AND SOFT DRINKS

Ginseng is now available in a wide variety of hair preparations, skin creams, and other beauty aids like the one my friend was devising in the 1970s. Ginseng has no value whatsoever in such products, and they usually only contain minute amounts anyway—just enough so that the manufacturer can put the name on the label to attract the gullible consumer. The same goes for most "ginseng" soft drinks.

MISNAMED "GINSENGS"

We saw in Chapter 13 that eleuthero root is sometimes misnamed "Siberian ginseng." The misnomer was invented by American marketing interests who wanted to piggyback this relatively inexpensive herb on the reputation of true Asian ginseng (*Panax ginseng*). Recently, I found a product labeled "Ginseng" in a supermarket. The ingredient-listing showed that it contained only eleuthero root. Several other tonic herbs are marketed in the U.S. today as "ginsengs," the term again being applied by marketing interests in order to improve the reputation of obscure herbs by association with the more familiar and highly valued Asian ginseng. Most such herbs have value as tonics and adaptogens, but generally do not compare to the potency or versatility of Asian ginseng.

True Ginsengs

Asian ginseng (*Panax ginseng*), American ginseng (*Panax quinquefolium*), tienchi ginseng (*Panax pseudoginseng*), and Japanese ginseng (*Panax japonicus*) are the only true ginsengs, being members of the same botanical genus and having similar, though not identical, properties. Japanese ginseng, considered by the Chinese to have weaker properties than Asian ginseng, is generally not available on the U.S. market. These ginsengs not only look much like Chinese ginseng, but they will even cross-pollinate with it. All these plants share some of the same ginsenosides and other constituents.

Second to eleuthero root, "Korean ginseng" is probably the most famous of the misnamed ginsengs, but Korean ginseng is true Asian ginseng, while eleuthero is not. Korean ginseng is actually *Panax ginseng*, but marketed by a Korean government agency. This misnomer is not an attempt to pass off another herb, but rather to develop the ginseng trade for Korean growers to compete with those in China. Korean ginseng is thus a brand name, not a plant name.

Around 1100 A.D., the Koreans did develop a new technique for preserving ginseng by steaming it and drying it in the sun. This produces a red-colored root, called *red* ginseng, that has stronger warming properties than unprocessed ginseng, which is called *white* ginseng. So "Korean *red* ginseng," a form widely available in products in the U.S., does indeed have slightly more stimulating properties than most ginseng from China. But the Koreans also market white ginseng, and the Chinese also produce steamed and sun-

Common name: Korean ginseng, Korean red ginseng
Latin name: *Panax ginseng*, same as Chinese ginseng
Uses: Same as for *Panax ginseng* in China
History: Knowledge of its use as a medicine introduced from China around the first century A.D. Most of the ginseng crop grown in Korea today originated from Chinese seed imported to that country after the Korean War.

dried red ginseng. I don't mention this to cast doubt on the quality of Korean ginseng products, which is usually high, but to dispel the misconception that "Korean ginseng" is a plant distinct from Chinese ginseng.

"Brazilian Ginseng"

Suma (*Pfaffia paniculata*) is regarded as a panacea in Brazil, much the way ginseng is in China. It has adaptogenic effects, and would probably be classified as a *chi* tonic in the Chinese system. It has some of the benefits of ginseng, including immune-stimulating, anti-cancer, hormone-regulating, and blood-sugar-regulating effects. The taste of suma is different from that of Chinese ginseng—it is more acrid than sweet—and it does not appear to have the warming properties of Chinese ginseng. Japanese researchers documented the tonic and adaptogenic properties of this plant, and it became available in U.S. stores in the late 1980s.

"Indian Ginseng"

Ashwaganda (*Withiania somnifera*) is held in high esteem in South Asia, similar to that of Chinese ginseng in China or suma in Brazil. Ashwaganda is the most famous tonic herb in Ayurvedic medicine, the traditional medicine of India. It is used to treat fatigue, general weakness, insomnia, the debility of old age, impotence, and infertility. It is more bitter and more warming than Chinese ginseng, and would be classified as a yang tonic in the Chinese system. Its presumed active constituents are entirely different than the ginsenosides and other constituents in the ginsengs. Ashwaganda has become more available in the U.S. over the last decade, as Ayurvedic medicine has grown in fame in this country.

American Red Ginseng

Some American ginseng roots grown in Michigan and Wisconsin are steam-cured the way Asian ginseng roots are cured in China and Korea. True wild American ginseng roots are never cured in this way, being of much higher value in their natural state. The problem is that the effects of curing on American ginseng are unknown. Steam-curing increases the warming properties of Chinese ginseng. The value of this practice with American roots is questionable because American ginseng's therapeutic value comes from its cooling and moistening properties. Steaming would presumably reduce these properties.

Another kind of "red ginseng" is an outright fraud. According to Michael Moore, Director of the Southwest School of Botanical Medicine in Albuquerque, New Mexico, and an expert on plants of the Southwest desert, some companies in the Southwest market a plant commonly known as caniagre (*Rumex hymenosepalus*) as an "American red desert ginseng," "Wild American red ginseng," or "Hymenosepalus ginseng." Caniagre has a natural reddish-brown color resembling that of cured ginseng. Caniagre has entirely different botanical and medicinal properties than ginseng, and possesses no adaptogenic effects.

Alaskan Ginseng

I've heard on the herbal grapevine that this new "ginseng" is about to appear on the market. The plant is actually Devil's Club (*Oplopanax horridum*). Like ginseng and eleuthero root, it is a member of the Aralia family. It was traditionally used by Native Americans to lower blood sugar levels in diabetics, something which ginseng will also do. Devil's Club has not been studied much by scientists. It will lower blood sugar levels, and probably has some adaptogenic effects, but a lot of study will be necessary before this plant can be marketed as an adaptogen. Russian researchers studied at least six of ginseng's cousins in the Aralia family, and of these found that only eleuthero root had adaptogenic properties.

CHAPTER 18

GINSENG PRODUCTS

Tonic herb products in the U.S. vary widely in both quality and price. In this chapter, I'll explain the various grades of Chinese and American ginseng, and tell how ginseng and other herbs are made into the products you might see in a store.

GINSENG ROOT GRADES

Whole Chinese and American ginseng roots come in a variety of grades carrying a wide range of prices. Here are the major grades of Chinese ginseng roots:

Wild *Tung Pei* Ginseng

Ginseng has been a popular and high-priced commodity in China for thousands of years. During that time, China has also suffered massive deforestation, depriving ginseng of its natural habitat. Thus, wild ginseng is now extremely rare in China. Perhaps only four or five pounds of it are discovered each year. A wild root can be up to 200 years old—older than most trees! Wild ginseng costs $500 to $600 a gram. That's about $15,000 an ounce, and more than $200,000 a pound. Finding such a root in China is the equivalent of winning the lottery. This grade is not for sale in the U.S. as a root, but both Dragon Eggs and Jade Chinese Herbals make products that contain a tiny amount of wild ginseng root.

Wild ginseng is renowned in Asia for its spiritual effects. A ginseng expert I know in the U.S. who practices meditation and *chi gong*, a Chinese practice that involves meditation on the *chi*, says that even four or five drops of an extract of wild ginseng root produces a noticeable spiritual high that lasts for days. This unusual property of wild roots may result from their long life. Most cultivated roots are harvested and sold when they are only four to six years old— infants, compared to the natural life span of ginseng. Wild roots are also occasionally found in Korea. These are also not available for sale in the U.S.

Yi Sun

Yi sun ginseng roots are called "semi-wild." They are grown from high-grade stock planted in a natural forest environment. The seedlings are allowed to grow for 8 to 12 years, and the resulting roots resemble wild ginseng. This is the most expensive grade available in the U.S. East Earth Tradewinds sells *Yi sun* roots by the gram. Prices vary as the market changes.

Shiu Chu

Shiu chu ginseng is widely available in the U.S. and is reasonably affordable. It can be purchased from East Earth

Tradewinds for $120 to $160 pound, which is the equivalent of about $3 to $7 a root, depending on size. The larger the root, the more valuable. *Shiu chu* ginseng is cultivated from selected superior ginseng stock. The roots are steamed and then cured in date sugar and other Chinese herbs, giving it a characteristic red color. If you are buying roots for regular use, I suggest that you get the highest grade—the largest size—of *Shiu chu* that you can find.

Kirin, Ji Lin

This cultivated ginseng is named after the region of China in which it is grown. Both are from Kirin province, the most important ginseng growing region in China. The cost of the ginseng roots cultivated there is about 75% that of *Shiu chu* ginseng. This is the lowest grade of ginseng, and the one found in most prepared ginseng products.

Grades by the Numbers

If you buy ginseng through catalogues or in stores, you will often see a number with the name, such as *Shiu Chu* 25, *Shiu Chu* 45, or *Kirin* #1 or #3. Ginseng is sold in China in lots of 1.3 pounds, called a *catty*. The number of roots it takes to make up the catty indicates the grade of the root. Since larger roots are more valuable, the lower number is a better grade. Thus, *Shiu Chu* 25 are larger and more valuable roots than *Shiu Chu* 45, because it takes only 25 roots to fill a catty instead of 45. The other grading system, #1, #2, #3, etc., works the opposite way. The #1 is a higher quality than the #2 or #3. Roots may also be of different sizes within each grade, graded as roots-per-catty or roots-per-pound. The fewer the roots-per-catty or pound, the better the quality and the higher the price.

AMERICAN GINSENG

Ginseng is becoming very scarce, and unless a method of cultivation becomes practical, bids fair to be exterminated.

Harvey Wickes Felter, M.D., 1898

In the century since Dr. Felter made the statement above, methods of cultivating ginseng have indeed become practical, and wild American ginseng remains on the verge of extinction. This would not be the case had the Native American method of harvesting the wild roots been adopted. Native Americans waited until the plant bore fruit, and then planted the seeds in the hole from which they dug the root, to ensure that the natural order would not be disturbed. A new method of growing ginseng—planting seedlings in the natural forest habitat—is a step closer to the Native American method, and has introduced a new quality of American ginseng to the market.

Wild Roots

American wild roots, although an endangered species, are not as rare as the Asian wild variety, and are not nearly as expensive. These are the highest-quality American ginseng roots. Like Asian ginseng, plants can live to be several hundred years old. Whether their medicinal superiority is enough to justify their higher price is questionable. The Chinese value wild-looking American roots for their appearance because of their similarity to the expensive wild Asian ginseng more than for their value as a medicine. This Chinese demand drives the price for wild American roots up unnaturally. Wild American ginseng roots are not for sale in stores or through catalogues, but must be purchased through commercial ginseng brokers. Because of their endangered status, some ethical companies are now using woods-grown semi-wild ginseng instead.

Woods-Grown

In the late 1980s, some growers began to plant seedlings in a natural forest habitat, much like the *Yi ʃun* ginseng of the Chinese. The roots began to mature within the last two years, and are now available through brokers and in some American products. Some growers use pesticides and fungicides on their woods-grown crop, just as large-scale ginseng farmers do. Others raise a completely organic product. Because genuine wild roots are so rare, and because of ethical problems surrounding their possible extinction, these organic woods-grown roots are the ones I recommend if you want to use American ginseng. They are superior in potency to cultivated roots.

Cultivated Roots

Ginseng cultivation began in earnest in the U.S. about 10 years after Dr. Felter made the statement predicting it. Most of the ginseng produced here is cultivated, with Michigan and Wisconsin being the biggest suppliers. American ginseng is the main cash crop in Marathon County, Wisconsin. Ginseng cultivation is expensive. It will only grow in the shade, so artificial structures must be erected to provide it. The cost of shade structures, planting, and cultivation is about $12,000 an acre. The plants must then grow for four to six years. In any year, the whole crop can be lost to fungus or other plant diseases, so agricultural chemicals are used extensively on the crops, increasing costs and yielding a product laced with fungicides and insecticides such as malathion. If you buy these roots, be sure to scrub them the way you would chemical-laced vegetables. The whole process is labor intensive, and by harvest time the roots have cost the farmer about $20 a pound. Ginseng can cost from 6 to 15 times that much by the time it reaches the consumer. About 95% of the annual crop of cultivated American ginseng is shipped to China.

This is the form of American ginseng most often available in stores or contained in commercial products. You can buy wild, woods-grown, or cultivated American ginseng from White Crane. Frontier Herb cooperative sells both woods-grown and cultivated American ginseng. East Earth Tradewinds and Spring Wind sell cultivated roots. Comparison-shop before making a purchase. HerbPharm sells an extract made from the organic woods-grown variety.

Red American Ginseng

Another development in recent years is steam-treating cultivated ginseng to make a red American ginseng like Korean and Chinese red products. This is a questionable practice, because steam-treatment of Chinese ginseng increases its warming properties. This would negate or moderate the valuable cooling property of American ginseng, its primary medical benefit.

CHINESE PREPARED FORMULAS

Chinese prepared formulas, called "patent formulas," are available in any Chinese store. They are appearing increasingly in health food stores. Thousands of these products exist. More than 250 companies in Beijing alone produce them. Many are based on classical Chinese formulas. The Chinese public purchases them the way Americans purchase over-the-counter remedies. Chinese medical practitioners usually prepare their own formulas from bulk herbs. They may also recommend patent formulas for minor conditions. Practitioners may also know how to sort the wheat from the chaff and identify high-quality prepared formulas. The patent formulas are usually in the form of small black pills or dark-colored liquids.

The quality of Chinese patent formulas is highly variable. They are usually made from the lowest grade of herbs; the higher quality herbs are sold to practitioners and the public in bulk. The patent formulas are proprietary products, and no one but the producers knows exactly what is in them or how they are made. The patents usually contain sugars and preservatives. Some have been found to contain potentially toxic heavy metals, which may be included in the formula intentionally or through contamination. Others have been found to contain strong Western drugs, such as steroids, that were not listed on the label.

Contamination with heavy metals, or the presence of drugs, is probably a minor problem, but poor-quality source material is very common. Some products, like the American ones I described in the last chapter, contain only minimal amounts of herbs. Tonic formulas, rather than formulas for acute conditions or pain relief, are the least likely to be contaminated. One brand of patent formulas made in China to the specification of American companies, without sugars or additives, is the Plum Flower Brand, available in stores or from K'an Herbals.

You need to know what you're doing before self-prescribing these patent formulas. Although they are balanced to prevent side effects, they can cause discomfort if you take the wrong formula for your condition. One book that describes these patent formulas and their medicinal actions is *Outline Guide to Chinese Herbal Patent Medicines in Pill Form*, by Margaret Naeser. It can be ordered from Boston Chinese Medicine at 617-720-4448.

AMERICAN PREPARED FORMULAS

With the rise of the profession of acupuncture and traditional Chinese medicine in the U.S. in the last 20 years, a new small industry has arisen to make high-quality products for these practitioners. Many of their products are available to consumers in stores or through mail order. The distinguishing characteristic of their products is that they are made from good-quality Chinese herbs. Like the Chinese patent medicines, these are based on classical Chinese formulas, sometimes modified to make them more appropriate for the American public, whose health problems differ somewhat from those of the Chinese. Since the early 1970s, the acupuncture profession in the U.S. has developed some of its own home-grown experts in traditional Chinese medicine. One, Dr. Ted Kaptchuk, is on the faculty of a division of Harvard Medical School. Kaptchuk has been a leader in modifying Chinese formulas for use by Americans.

Liquid Extracts

Many of the companies mentioned above make concentrated liquid extracts of formulas. They prepare an herbal
formula similarly to the way you would make a tonic tea, as
I described in Chapter 15. Sometimes water or alcohol, or
both, is used to extract the constituents from the herbs. The
resulting product is concentrated to make a potent liquid
extract. A dropperful of such an extract might contain the
same constituents you would get from one or two cups of
a tea.

Most liquid herbal products that you see in stores are
tinctures: simple, unconcentrated extracts in water and
alcohol. The liquid extracts I refer to are much more potent
than tinctures. I have felt a stronger effect from 12-drop
doses of one high-quality ginseng extract prepared in this
way than I have ever felt from the tea of a low-grade cultivated root. An advantage of liquid extracts is that they are
very digestible; all of the fibrous, hard-to-digest constituents
of the plant have been removed.

Pills and Capsules

Some companies also make products that are simple
mixtures of powdered herbs. More often, though, the pills
and capsules are made from the extracts I described above.
The solvent is evaporated to leave a gummy residue which is
then mixed with an inert binding material to make the pill or
capsule. This form is very potent, and, like the liquid extract,
is easy to assimilate.

Granules

Other companies sell Chinese herbal products in granule form. A tea is prepared in the usual way, although in a large vat instead of in a pot on your stove. The water is then evaporated, and the residue is made into dissolvable granules. Some acupuncturists use these granules instead of bulk herbs because the granules are easy to mix, and because the patient will not have to go to the bother of brewing a messy tea. All you have to do is add the granules to a cup of hot water. These granules are not generally available to the public, being restricted to practitioner use.

Tinctures

Some American companies, mostly those unfamiliar with Chinese herbalism, make simple tinctures of Chinese herbs. A typical concentration is one part of the herb to five parts of solvent (1:5 on the label). The Chinese do not use herbs this way, and thus it is difficult to know what a proper dose would be. This method is used in the West for herbs that require low doses for medicinal activity. The Chinese, on the other hand, prefer larger doses, especially of the tonic herbs. To get a sufficient dose from such a simple tincture could be prohibitively expensive. I recommend the more concentrated extracts from companies that specialize in Chinese herbs.

CHAPTER 19

OVERVIEW

In this chapter, I'll review the indications for ginseng and the tonic herbs, and suggest some herbal therapies you might try if you have an excess condition and cannot take the tonics. Chinese medicine has treatments for excess, but there's no reason to turn to China when Western herbalism offers so many simple and inexpensive therapies.

THE ALTERATIVE HERBS

In Chapter 4, I showed you how to distinguish among excess, deficient, hot, and cold conditions. Conditions of excess are common in Americans, and Western herbal therapy excels in treating them with a class of herbs known in Western traditions as alteratives (from the word "to alter"). They are also called "tonics" in Western herbalism. Although the name is the same, these herbs have nothing in common with the Chinese tonics. Western herbalism was developed on a population of robust peasants and farmers who were generally well fed and prone to conditions of excess—the constitutional opposite of many Chinese people.

243

TABLE 19.1
HERBAL THERAPIES AND LIFESTYLE
CHANGES FOR THE SIX CONDITIONS

	Excess	Deficient
Hot	Tonics not appropriate	American ginseng Yin tonics Blood tonics
	Alterative herbs Burdock Dandelion root Stinging Nettles Yellow dock	Other ginsengs and *chi* and yang tonics contra- indicated
	Juice fasting Vegetarian diet or reduce meat intake No junk food No stimulants	Moistening, nourishing herbs Slippery elm, marshmallow root Absolutely no stimulants
	Moderate aerobic exercise	Fruits, soups, beverage herb teas Chrysanthemum tea Light exercise (walking in nature) Meditation and rest
Cold	Tonics not appropriate	Asian ginseng Red ginseng Siberian ginseng

Alteratives will restore a system that is thrown out of balance through too much heat or accumulated food and toxins. Take alterative herbs for three to six weeks, rather than short-term like a cold remedy or an antacid.

TABLE 19.1 *continued*

	Excess	Deficient
Cold (*cont.*)	Warming digestive herbs	*Chi* tonics
		Yang tonics
	Warm meals, soups	Blood tonics
	Smaller, more frequent meals	Cooling herbs contraindicated
	Screen for allergenic foods	
		Digestive herbs if needed
	No junk food	for poor digestion or
	No dairy products	malabsorption
		No stimulants
	Aerobic exercise according to capacity	Nourishing foods; screen for allergenic foods
		Light, enjoyable exercise
Interior	Tonics not appropriate	Tonics selected according to factors of heat or cold, as in column above
Exterior	Tonics not appropriate	Tonics contraindicated without first resolving the acute condition (cold, flu, allergy attack)

The pathology of an excess condition is this: the individual may overeat, or eat foods that are too heavy and hard to digest. Farmers who put in 10 or 12 hours of heavy labor a day may be able to get away with this, but most of us can't.

Lack of exercise makes the condition worse. The digestive system becomes overloaded and worn out, and the liver becomes stagnant. The composition of the blood becomes deranged due to the sluggish action of the liver. The eliminative organs also become overloaded, and undigested food builds up in the digestive tract. Toxins accumulate throughout the system, and the individual becomes susceptible to a wide variety of diseases. Atherosclerosis and coronary heart disease are common manifestations of this pathology.

The sixteenth-century physician Paracelsus described one result of these conditions as "tartaric diseases," after the tartaric sediment that collects at the bottom of a wine barrel. The "sediments" in an excess individual may manifest as gall stones, kidney stones, arthritic inflammation of the joints, or allergies if the sediments collect in the soft tissues. Paracelsus said that there was one cause of such diseases: too much food. A person in such condition may feel sluggish, weak, and depressed, but this is not the weakness of deficiency. Turn-of-the-century books on medical herbalism described the strategy for treating such conditions: "Improve the nutrition and increase the wastes."

Improve the Nutrition

The strategy for improving the nutrition is two-fold. If you have an excess condition, you will have to adjust your diet.

Two of the most famous Western naturopathic dietary treatments — vegetarianism and fasting — were developed for people with excess conditions or constitutions. You needn't become completely vegetarian or undertake extreme fasts to improve your condition; the vegetables are the most important part of the treatment. A three-day vegetable fast, eating only vegetables, once a month may be helpful.

When I was attending a naturopathic medical college, I heard of another variation: eat five pounds of vegetables a day for a week. The doctor describing this diet quipped that the patient could eat whatever else they wanted that they had room for after eating the vegetables. Five pounds of vegetables is the same weight as twenty quarter-pounder hamburgers, and a lot more bulky. Periodic fasting on fresh-made vegetable juices and vegetable broths may also help. Books on fasting are available in most health food stores. This all-but-forgotten healing technique is extremely valuable for restoring an excess constitution to health.

As a minimum, cut down on meat intake and increase the vegetable and whole-grain portion of your diet. Cut out junk food and fast food as much as possible. Let half of each meal be fruits and vegetables. People with hot excess conditions can eat their vegetables either cooked or raw. Make a meal of a large salad, emphasizing solid vegetables over iceberg lettuce, which is an "empty" and unsatisfying food with little nutritional value. If you have a cold excess condition, eat the vegetables cooked, with some warming spices such as curry, ginger, cardamom, chilies, and so on.

Herbal remedies can also provide nutrition, and they fall into two general categories: bitter tonics, and warming digestive stimulants.

Bitter Tonics   Herbs with a bitter flavor increase digestive secretions and stimulate the liver to secrete bile. They are ideal for people with hot, excess constitutions, though they should not be used during an episode of pain in the digestive tract, such as heartburn.

Goldenseal   The most famous of these herbs is goldenseal (*Hydrastis canadensis*). Goldenseal is often used in the U.S. today to treat colds and flu. About half the people who use it misuse it; it is best for a cold with heat signs and a runny nose, especially a yellow mucous discharge. Goldenseal is not appropriate for a "dry" cold with chilly feelings. Herbalist physicians of the last century used goldenseal as one of their premier bitter tonics to restore digestion in run-down, excess constitutions. If you want to take goldenseal as a tonic, I suggest that you use low doses: 20 drops of a tincture or a single capsule of powder, broken open and stirred into a cup of warm water. Take it 10 minutes before meals, on an empty stomach. Goldenseal tea is not as effective, because some constituents are not soluble in water and the root material gets discarded with the tea.

Oregon Grape Root   Oregon grape root (*Berberis aquifolium*) is closely related to goldenseal, and shares some of the same bitter constituents. You can take it the same way. Oregon grape root is much less expensive than goldenseal. You might also prefer it because goldenseal is becoming endangered through over-harvesting in its natural habitat.

Gentian   This is the most famous of the European bitter tonics. It is included in many of the digestive bitter drinks that are popular as a pre-meal appetizer in Europe. You can purchase digestive bitters like the European ones in most health food stores. A half-and-half mixture of powdered gentian and ginger is a common remedy in naturopathic medicine, where it is used as a tonic for people with excess conditions.

SOME ALTERATIVE HERBS FOR EXCESS CONSTITUTIONS

Stronger tonics

Goldenseal	*Hydrastis canadensis*
Oregon grape root	*Berberis aquifolium*
Gentian	*Gentiana lutea*
Barberry	*Berberis vulgaris*

Milder tonics

Yellow dock	*Rumex crispus*
Burdock root	*Arctium lappa*
Dandelion root	*Taraxacum officinalis*

Alterative diuretics

Juniper berries	*Juniperus officinalis*
Stinging nettle	*Urtica dioica*
Dandelion leaf	*Taraxacum officinalis*

Milder Bitter Herbs   The above herbs have a strong bitter taste, and a strong immediate action on the system. See the following box for a list of milder bitters. These are better overall alteratives because they have more wide-ranging effects on the system. All improve digestion, liver function, and nutrition, but burdock and dandelion also have mild diuretic effects and help to decrease excess fluids. Yellow dock has a mild laxative effect and improves bowel function. Use doses of yellow dock similar to those for the stronger bitter tonics. Burdock and dandelion may be taken in larger doses, and make wonderful tea. They can be consumed like coffee, three cups a day. These are two of my top ten favorite herbs, among those that I prescribe most often. Take them for three to six weeks, then break for a week or two.

Increase Quantity of the Wastes

The above tonics all aid in the elimination of excess in a variety of ways. They stimulate the action of the liver to secrete bile, which is a natural laxative. The improved liver function will also help purify the blood; the liver is the physiological equivalent of the oil filter in your car.

Constipation   If you are constipated (a common symptom of an excess constitution with deficient digestion), I recommend against taking laxatives. The high-vegetable diet above, warm water with a little lemon added, and alterative herbs will usually do the job by correcting the cause rather than by artificially stimulating the bowels. Many laxatives can also create laxative dependence. Of the herbs above, yellow dock has the most laxative activity.

Diuretic Alteratives   Some alteratives promote kidney function and promote elimination of excess fluids through that organ. Juniper berries are excellent for this purpose, and also have bitter tonic qualities for the digestive tract. They also contain warming volatile oils, and thus are suitable for conditions of cold and excess.

The famous German nature-cure healer and herbalist, Father Sebastian Kneipp, gave juniper berries to patients reluctant to undergo his full regimen of fasting, dietary changes, and hydrotherapy. He would give them a large bag of juniper berries, and tell them to eat 5 the first day, 6 the second, 7 the third, and so on, until they were taking 30 berries a day. He would then have them taper the dose by 1 berry a day until they were back to 5 a day. Kneipp said that after doing this, the patients invariably felt so much better that they would then submit to his entire method of cure. Juniper berries stimulate the digestion, improve liver function, and promote elimination of fluid accumulations. You can also take 20 drops of juniper berry tincture three times a day.

Stinging nettle is another of my top ten herbs. It is highly nutritive, and also diuretic. Take it as a tea, two or three cups a day. Capsules are also available in health food stores. Dandelion greens have an action similar to dandelion root on the liver and digestive tract, but are also a strong diuretic. One animal trial found that dandelion leaf was comparable in potency to the pharmaceutical diuretic furosemide (Lasix). Take dandelion leaf as a tea, or pick the greens from your yard or a field in the spring (avoid any where pesticides may be used), and cook them in stir-fries or soups. The younger greens are not so bitter, but the older ones can be quite unpalatable. You can simmer them in a little water for 5 to 10 minutes, then pour the water off to reduce the bitter taste.

COLD CONDITIONS

Cold excess conditions may be treated with the above dietary methods and the milder herbs, but you'll need to add warming spices and herbs. Cooked vegetables with warming spices are medicine for this condition. The most important dietary changes are to cut down on dairy foods (no ice cream!), junk food, fast food, and overeating in general. Add fennel seed or ginger to your alterative tea, or mix the herb powders with 50% ginger root powder. Take a mild ginger root tea (get the whole roots in a grocery store) with lemon and a little honey as a daily beverage. The digestive tea I described in Chapter 14 is well suited to either hot or cold conditions of excess with deficient digestion.

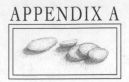

Where to Buy Ginseng and the Tonic Herbs

GINSENG ROOTS are hard to find unless you have access to an Asian store. In this appendix, I'll tell you where to order ginseng roots and other bulk tonic herbs by mail. I'll also describe some of the American companies that make high-quality Chinese tonic formulas. Most of these companies make their products for the professional acupuncturist or herbalist markets, but they also sell products through health food stores or directly to consumers through the mail. This is by no means a complete list of such companies, so please don't think that, because a particular company is not listed, its products are in any way inferior.

GINSENG ROOTS AND BULK HERBS

Chinese and American ginseng roots in a variety of grades are available from the following companies:

East Earth Tradewinds
P.O. Box 493151
Redding, CA 96049-3151
800-258-6878
Fax: 800-258-1384
East Earth Tradewinds sells all grades of ginseng root except true wild Chinese ginseng. They carry several grades of *Kirin*, several grades of *Shiu Chu*, and semi-wild *Yi Sun* ginseng. East Earth will sell the roots by the ounce, which is an advantage over some other suppliers who require purchases of a half-pound or a pound. They also sell American ginseng roots by the ounce. A full line of Chinese tonic herbs are available in $\frac{1}{4}$- and $\frac{1}{2}$-pound quantities. If you only want to get one catalog, this is the one for you. They also distribute formulas by a number of companies, including Dragon Eggs, Jade Chinese Herbals, Imperial Elixir, McZand Herbal Supplements, and some of the formulas by herbalist Ron Teeguarden that I've described in this book. You can also order Chinese patent formulas, herbal products for martial artists, books, and tea-making supplies, including the ginseng cooker I described in Chapter 15.

Spring Wind
2315 Fourth Street
Berkeley, CA 94710
510-849-1820
800-588-4883 (orders)
Fax: 510-859-4886
Spring Wind has the widest assortment of Chinese herbs and the best prices of all the companies I list here. They usually sell only to medical practitioners, but will sell ginseng and other tonic herbs to consumers. You may have to order using the Chinese or Latin names of the herbs. Spring Wind sells several grades of ginseng root as well as sliced roots, which are much less expensive than whole roots. They also sell different sizes of cultivated American ginseng roots.

White Crane
426 First Street
Jersey City, NJ 07302

800-994-3721
Internet: crane@inch.com
White Crane sells all varieties and sizes of American ginseng roots. They will sell in lots as small as a quarter pound. American-grown fresh Chinese herbs and other fresh Western herbs are also a specialty.

Frontier Herb Cooperative
P.O. Box 299
Norway, IA 52318
800-717-4372
Frontier is primarily a distributor of Western bulk herbs, spices, and herb products, and is one of the largest in the country. They also sell Chinese and American ginseng in several grades, as well as some of the tonic herbs described in Chapter 13. Their prices are high for Chinese herbs, compared to the sources above; they are about what you would find in a retail store.

PROFESSIONAL-LEVEL TONIC FORMULAS

Crane Enterprises
45 Samoset Ave
Plymouth, MA 02360
800-227-4118
Crane Enterprises sells a wide variety of prepared tonic formulas, including those made by K'an Herbals, Health Concerns, and others.

East Earth Herb, Inc.
P.O. Box 2802
Eugene, OR 97402
800-827-4372
Fax: 503-485-7347
East Earth Herbs is the producer and manufacturer of the Jade Chinese Herbals line, which I've described in several places in the book. They produce a top line of tonic formulas. East Earth also formulates and produces products for many other companies, and has a reputation for high ethical standards and excellent products.

Gaia Herbs
62 Old Littleton Road
Harvard, MA 01451
800-831-7780
Fax: 800-717-1722
GAIA primarily sells high-quality Western herbal tinctures. Their concentrated ginseng extracts and Chinese liquid formulas are among the best available.

Health Concerns
8001 Capwell Drive
Oakland, CA 94621
510-639-0280 (herbal help line)
800-233-9355
Health Concerns makes its own line of herbal formulas, including tonics. The formulas are based on traditional Chinese blends, and modified by clinical experts from China and the U.S. Health Concerns also distributes products made by other companies, including Seven Forests, Turtle Mountain, McZand, and K'an. Also available are books, audiotapes, and a newsletter.

HerbPharm
P.O. Box 116
Williams, OR 97544
800-348-4372
HerbPharm has a reputation as one of the most ethical of the Western herbal tincture companies. Their Asian ginseng, American ginseng, and eleuthero root concentrated extracts are among the best available.

Institute for Traditional Medicine
2017 S.E. Hawthorne
Portland, OR 97214
800-544-7504
Fax: 503-233-1017
The Institute for Traditional Medicine (ITM) sells a large number of prepared formulas and educational materials. They produce the Seven

Forests line of formulas, one of the most innovative in tailoring traditional formulas specifically to the needs of Americans. A reference book available from ITM, *A Bag of Pearls*, describes the composition and medicinal uses of each formula, including the tonic formulas.

The ITM also sells products made by Health Concerns, and a number of Chinese patent formulas.

K'an Herb Company
6001 Butler Lane
Scotts Valley, CA 95066
800-543-5233
Fax: 408-438-9457
K'an produces product lines called K'an Herbals, Chinese Modular Solutions, and K'an Herbal Traditional. They also sell products made by Health Concerns, and a number of Chinese patent medicines, including the quality Plum Flower brand. Books are also available.

McZand Herbal, Inc.
P.O. Box 5312
Santa Monica, CA 90409
310-822-0500
McZand produces the Zand Formulas line, which is available in many health food stores. They also produce products for practitioners, including high-quality extracts of single herbs and tonic formulas. The consumer line includes some excellent tonics, including the formula devised for the athletes at the 1984 Summer Olympics in Los Angeles. The professional line includes some excellent tonic products based on traditional Chinese formulas. McZand won't sell their professional line directly to consumers, but the tonic formulas may be ordered through East Earth or Health Concerns.

Turtle Island Herbs
412 Boulder Street
Boulder, CO 80302
303-442-2215
Turtle Island makes a top-quality American ginseng tincture and a full line of organic and wild-crafted Western herb tinctures.

Wise Woman Herbals
P.O. Box 279
Creswell, OR 97426
800-532-5219
Wise Woman Herbals offers a full-line of high-quality tinctures of
Western herbs including American ginseng.

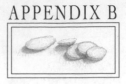

Where to Find a Practitioner of Natural Medicine

To find a licensed practitioner of Oriental medicine, try the following referral resource:

American Association of Acupuncture and Oriental Medicine
433 Front Street
Catasauqua, PA 18032
610-433-2448

The AAAOM maintains a database of more than six thousand licensed practitioners in the U.S. They will give you over the phone the names of a few practitioners near you, or will send you a printout of all the practitioners in your state.

The AAAOM database can provide information about the level of training and education of each practitioner. The education for licensure focuses mostly on acupuncture, with only a basic education in Chinese herbalism. Some acupuncturists go on to get more education in herbalism, either through seminars, course work, or self-study, and take a certification exam for herbalism. I suggest that you ask for a referral to a practitioner who has passed the "NCCA Herbalist Exam."

The database can also tell the conditions that the practitioners treat. If you have a particular chronic condition, be sure to ask ahead of time for a practitioner who can treat it.

OTHER ALTERNATIVE PRACTITIONERS

American Association of Naturopathic Physicians
2366 Eastlake Avenue East
Suite #322
Seattle, WA 98102
206-323-7610

American College of Advancement in Medicine
P.O. Box 3427
Laguna Hills, CA 92654
714-583-7666

Canadian Association of Ayurvedic Medicine
P.O. Box 749 Station B
Ottawa, Ontario
Canada K1P 5P8

INFORMATION ABOUT HERBAL MEDICINE

American Botanical Council
P.O. Box 201660
Austin, TX 78720-1660
512-331-8868

Herb Research Foundation
1007 Pearl Street
Suite #200
Boulder, CO 80302
800-748-2617

PUBLICATIONS

HerbalGram
(Order through the American Botanical Council)
HerbalGram covers regulatory news, scientific reviews, features, and other topics of interest on herbs. It is the joint newsletter of the American Botanical Council and the Herb Research foundation. Herbal-Gram has an extensive list of herbal textbooks available for order through the mail.

Medical Herbalism
P.O. Box 33080
Portland, OR 97233
303 541-9552
A quarterly clinical newsletter aimed at practitioners, but an important resource for any student of herbal healing.

APPENDIX C
TONIC HERBS AND THEIR ACTIONS

| Herb | Type of tonic | | | | Chinese Organs Affected | | | | | | Temp. |
	chi	blood	yang	yin	Spleen	Stomach	Lung	Liver	Heart	Kidney	w=warm c=cool n=neutral
Asian ginseng	●	○		○	●		●				w
American ginseng	○			●			●		○	○	c
Antler	○	○	●					●		●	w
Asparagus				●		●	●			●	c
Astragalus	●				●		●				w
Atractylodes	●				●						w
Codonopsis	●			○	●	●	●				n
Cordyceps			●	●			●			●	n
Dendrobium				●			●			●	c
Dioscorea	●		○	○	●		●			●	n
Dong quai		●		○				●			w
Eleuthero	●		●		●				●	●	w
Eucommia			●	●				●		●	w
Fo Ti		●						●		●	w
Ganoderma	●				●		○	○	●	○	w
Glehnia				●		●	●				c
Jujube date	●			○	●	●			●		n

continued

Herb	Type of tonic				Chinese Organs Affected						Temp. (w=warm, c=cool, n=neutral)
	chi	blood	yang	yin	Spleen	Stomach	Lung	Liver	Heart	Kidney	
Licorice	●				●	○	●	○	○	○	n
Ligustrum				●				●		●	n
Lycium		●		●				●		●	n
Morindae			●					●		●	w
Peony		●		●	●			●			c
Poria	○			○	●		●	●			n
Prince ginseng	●			●	●		●		●		n
Rehmannia		●				●		●	●	●	w
Royal jelly	●	●							●		n
Schizandra							●		●	●	w
Tienchi ginseng	●					●		●			w
Citrus peel					●	●	●				w
Ginger					●	●	●			●	w
Ligusticum								●			w
Bupleurum								●			c

Adjuvant herbs used in formulas to enhance the effects of tonic herbs

● means primary effect, ○ is secondary effect

BIBLIOGRAPHY

Beinfield, Harriet and Efrem Korngold. *Between Heaven and Earth: A Guide to Chinese Medicine.* New York: Ballantine Books, 1991.

Bensky, Dan and Andrew Gamble. *Chinese Herbal Medicine Materia Medica.* Seattle: Eastland Press, 1986.

Bensky, Dan and Randall Barolet. *Formulas and Strategies.* Seattle: Eastland Press, 1990.

Bergner, Paul. "Ginseng abuse: a case study" *Medical Herbalism.* 8(1):14-15, 1986

Chen, Ze-lin and Chen Mei-fang. *A Comprehensive Guide to Chinese Herbal Medicine.* Long Beach, California: Oriental Healing Arts Institute, 1992.

Coulter, Harris. *Divided Legacy* (four volumes). Washington, D.C.: Center for Empirical Medicine, 1986.

Dharmananda, S. *The Ginseng Story.* Portland, OR: Institute for Traditional Medicine, 1994.

Farnsworth, N.R. Personal communication, January 29, 1991. Cited in *The Honest Herbal* (Third Edition), by Varro E. Tyler. New York: Haworth Press, 1993.

Felter, H.W. and Ju Lloyd. *King's American Dispensatory.* Portland, OR: Eclectic Medical Publications, 1983. [Reprinted from 1898 original].

Foster, S. *Asian Ginseng:* Panax ginseng. Austin, Texas: American Botanical Council, 1991.

Foster, S. *American Ginseng:* Panax quinquefolium. Austin, Texas: American Botanical Council, 1991.

Foster, S. *Herbal Emissaries.* Rochester, Vermont: Healing Arts Press, 1992.

Fratkin, Jake Paul. *Chinese Classics: Popular Chinese Herbal Formulas*. Santa Fe, New Mexico: SHYA Publications, 1990.

Fulder, Stephen. *Ginseng and Other Chinese Herbs for Vitality*. Rochester, Vermont: Healing Arts Press, 1980.

Hardacre, Val. *Woodland Nuggets of Gold*. Northville, Michigan: Holland House Press, 1968.

Harding, A.R. *Ginseng and Other Medicinal Plants*. Columbus, Ohio: A.R. Harding. Revised edition, 1972.

Hobbs, Christopher. *Medicinal Mushrooms*. Santa Cruz, California; Botanica Press, 1995.

Hsu, Hong-yen. *Oriental Materia Medica: A Concise Guide*. New Canaan, Connecticut: Keats Publishing, 1986.

Hu, S.Y. "Knowledge of Ginseng from Chinese Records." *Journal of the Chinese University of Hong Kong*. 4(2):283–305, 1977.

Kaptchuk, Ted. *The Web That Has No Weaver: Understanding Chinese Medicine*. New York: Congden and Weed, 1983.

Lee, F.C. *Facts About Ginseng: The Elixir of Life*. Elizabeth, New Jersey: Hollym International Corp., 1992.

Leung, Albert Y. *Chinese Herbal Remedies*. New York: Phaedon Universe, 1984.

Naeser, Margaret. *Outline Guide to Chinese Herbal Patent Medicines in Pill Form*. Boston, Massachusetts: Boston Chinese Medicine, 1990.

Ni, Maoshing. *Chinese Herbology Made Easy*. Los Angeles: College of Tao and Traditional Chinese Healing, 1986.

Osol, Arthur, et al. *The Dispensatory of the United States of America*. Philadelphia: J.B. Lippencott Company, 1947.

Schauenberg, P., and Ferdinand Paris. *Guide to Medicinal Plants*. New Canaan, Connecticut: Keats Publishing, 1977.

Siegel, R.K. "Ginseng abuse syndrome" *Journal of the American Medical Association*. 241:1614-1615, 1979; 243:32, 1980.

Teeguarden, Ron. *Chinese Herbs*. Tokyo and New York: Japan Pulications, 1984.

Tierra, Michael. *Planetary Herbology*. Santa Fe: Lotus Press, 1988.

Tyler, Varro E. *The Honest Herbal* (Third Edition). New York: Haworth Press, 1993.

Wiseman, Nigel and Andrew Ellis. *Fundamentals of Chinese Medicine*. Brookline, Massachusetts: Paradigm Publications, 1985.

INDEX

Joint pain, 47
Journal of the American Medical Association, 77
Jujube dates, 35, 53–54, 83, 134, 141, 145, 147, 158, 169–170
In athletic formula, 211
Juniper berries, 249
Juniperus off., 249

K'an Herbals, 142, 179
Kashuu, 166
Kidney, 30, 52, 57–59, 143, 146, 154–155, 156, 158, 163, 164, 165, 174, 178, 180
Kidney deficiency, symptom list, 133
Kidney disease, 170
Korea, 8
Korean Ginseng Research Institute, 109

Lactate, 95, 207
Lafitau, Joseph Francois, 9
Large Intestine, 52, 181
Lawrence Review of Natural Products, 104
Laxative properties, 167
Learning, 99–100
Lee, Florence C., 109
Lethargy, 21, 23, 44
Leung, Albert Y., 111
Licorice, 54, 66, 136, 141, 149–151, 153, 155, 170–173, 176, 181, 183, 201
In athletic formula, 210–211, 216
Lifestyle, 18, 32–40
Lifestyle Chinese vs. American, table, 38
Ligusticum, 136, 167, 175, 184
Ligustrum, 148–149, 158, 173
Ligustrum lucidum. See Ligustrum
Ling Zhi Feng Wang Jiang, 179
Ling zhi, 167
Lips, pale, 24
Liver, 52, 56–57, 100, 156, 164–165, 174–175, 178–179, 181, 184
See also Hepatoprotectant
Liver deficiency. Symptom list, 133
Liver disease, 171
Locoweed, 147

Longevity, 4–5, 93
Low back pain, 58
Lu rong. See Deer antler
Lung, 52, 55–56, 141, 143, 146–147, 151–152, 154–156, 169–170, 176–177, 180
Lung chi, 74
Lung deficiency. Symptom list, 132
Lycium berry, 146–147, 154, 158, 174–175, 180–181
In athletic formula, 216
Lycium chinensis. See Lycium berry

Ma huang, 124–125
Contraindication for Asian ginseng, 79
Malt sugar, 149
Manchuria, 4
McZand Herbals, 135–136, 150
Medicine, Arabic, 37
Medicine, Ayurvedic. *See* Ayurveda, 27
Medicine, Chiropractic, 26
Medicine, constitutional. *See* Constitution
Medicine, conventional, 25
Medicine, naturopathic, 26, 31
Meditation, 64
Medvedev, M.A., 104
Memory, poor, 24
Menopause, 100–101, 179
Menses, excessive. Contraindication for Asian ginseng, 79
Menstrual disorders, 12–13, 24, 54, 79, 157, 171, 175, 178, 182
Mental activity, 21, 23
Meridians, 19
Metabolic effects, 90, 101
Mongols, 8
Morinda off. See Morindae
Morindae, 174–175
In athletic formula, 214
Motion sickness, 183
Movement, voluntary, 21, 23
Mucous, excess, 165, 178
Muscle pain, 47
Muscle weakness, 54
Muscles, 21–23, 175

ABOUT THE AUTHOR

Paul Bergner is the editor of *Medical Herbalism* and *Clinical Nutrition Update*, and clinic director at the Rocky Mountain Center for Botanical Studies in Boulder, Colorado. He was the founding editor of *The Naturopath Physician* magazine, has contributed articles to *The Townsend Letter for Doctors*, and has been a contributing editor for *Natural Health*, *The Nutrition and Dietary Consultant*, and *Health World*. In addition to his chapters in *American Herbalism: Essays on Herbs and Herbalism* by Members of the American Herbalists Guild, he is co-author of *Safety, Effectiveness, and Cost Effectiveness in Naturopathic Medicine* and author of *Twelve Powerful Herbs*, and *The Healing Power of Garlic*.